FIGHTING THE FAMINE

First published in 1985 by Pluto Press Limited,
The Works, 105a Torriano Avenue, London NW5 2RX
and Pluto Press Australia Limited, PO Box 199, Leichhardt,
New South Wales 2040, Australia

7 6 5 4 3 2 1

89 88 87 86 85

Designed by Roger Huddle
Set by Kate Macpherson Photosetting, Clevedon, Avon
Printed in Great Britain by BAS Printers Limited,
Over Wallop, Stockbridge, Hampshire SO20 8JD
Bound by W. H. Ware & Sons Limited, Tweed Road, Clevedon, Avon

British Library Cataloguing in Publication Data
Twose, Nigel
    Fighting the famine
    1. Africa — Famines
    I. Title
    363.8   HC800.Z9F3

ISBN 0 7453 0131 2

Pluto 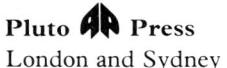 **Press**
London and Sydney

FIGHTING THE FAMINE

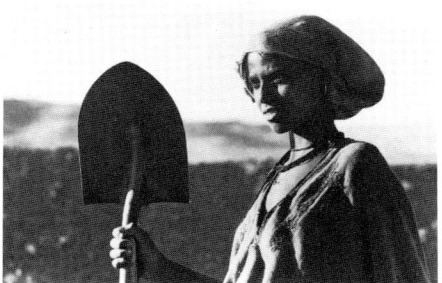

Text by Nigel Twose ● Photographs by Mike Goldwater

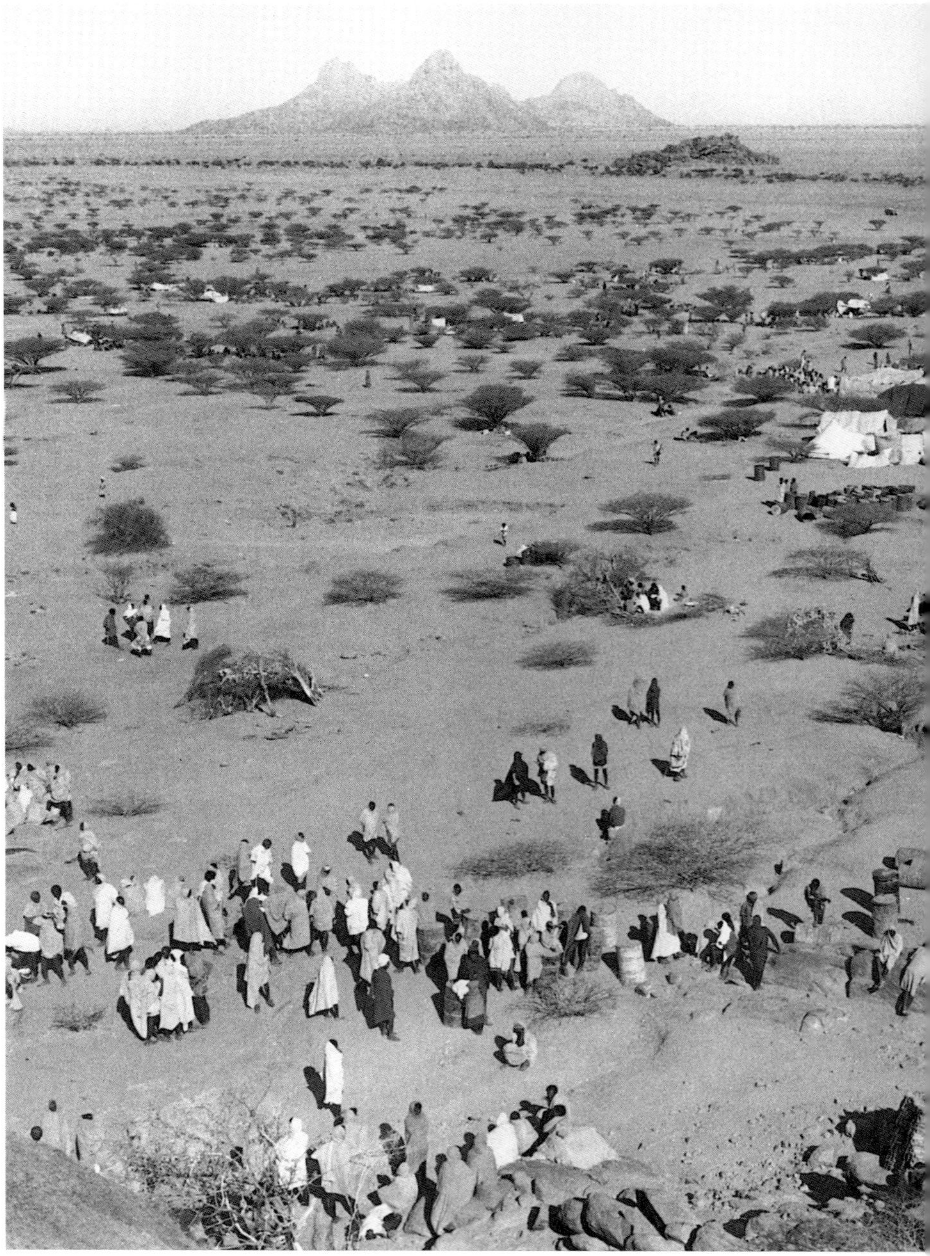

4

Acknowledgements

Our thanks to Wendy Wallace for her editing of the text, and to the aid agencies listed on page 95 for their support for the project.

CONTENTS

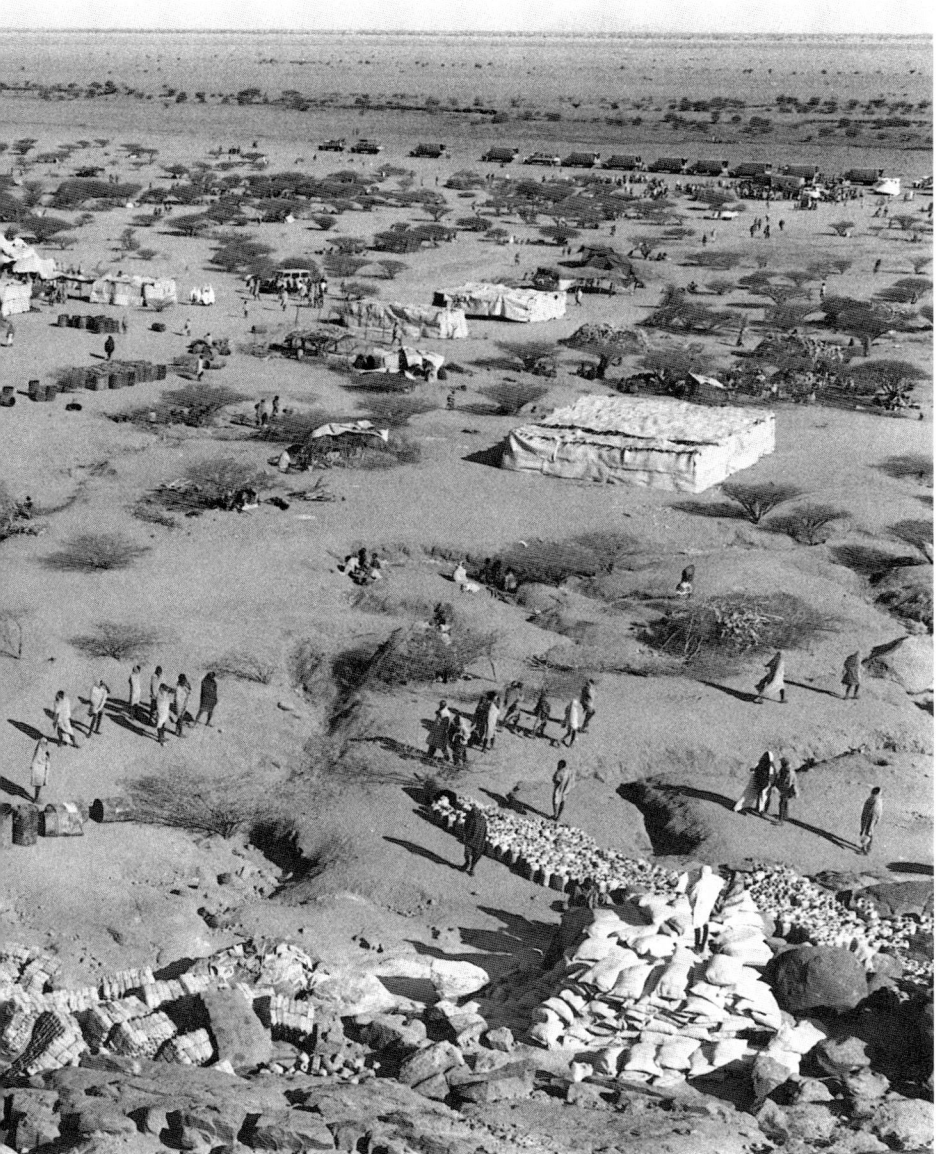

5

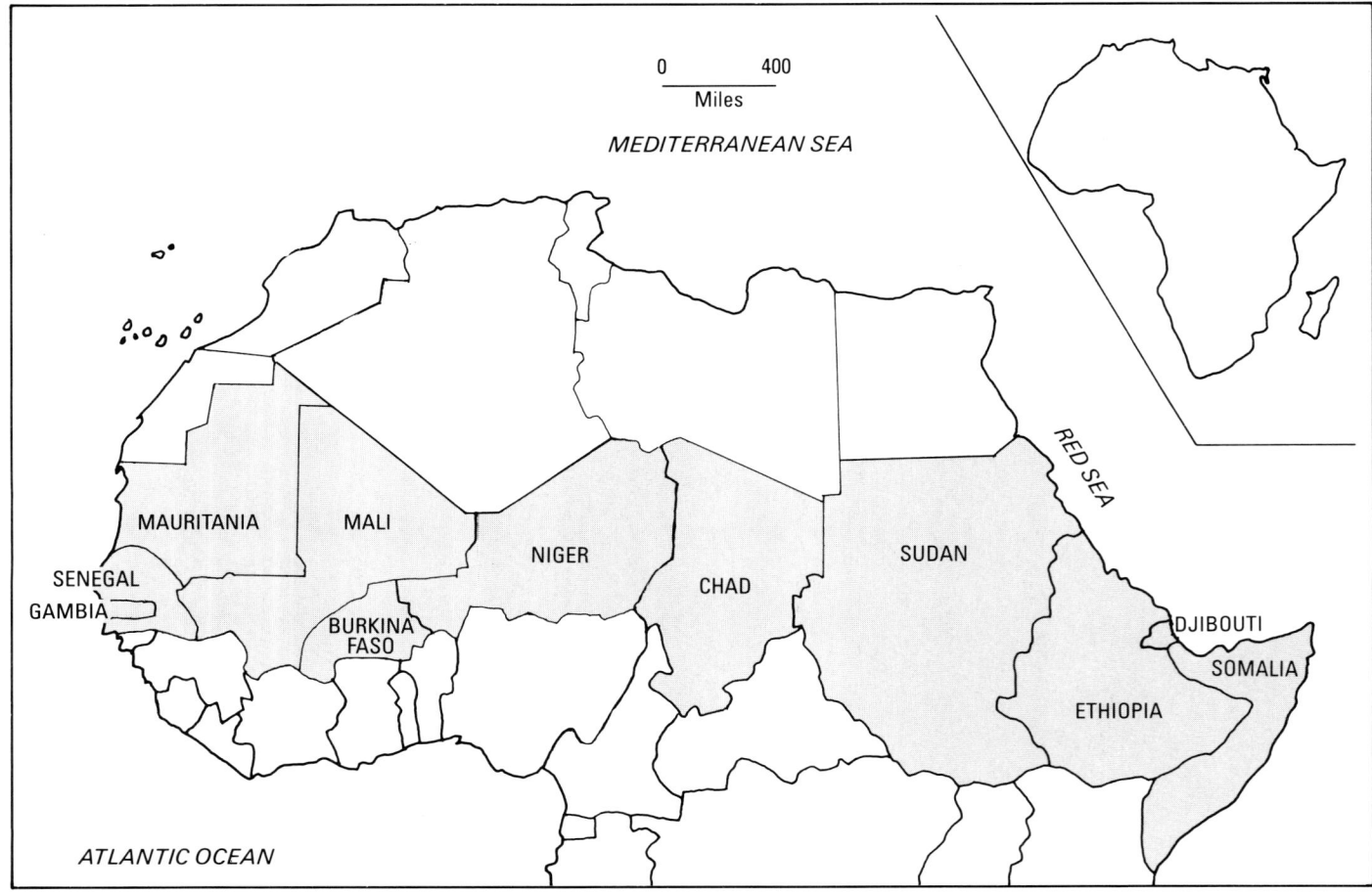

MEDITERRANEAN SEA

0   400
Miles

RED SEA

MAURITANIA

MALI

NIGER

SUDAN

SENEGAL

GAMBIA

CHAD

DJIBOUTI

BURKINA
FASO

SOMALIA

ETHIOPIA

ATLANTIC OCEAN

**All the countries shaded on the map are
those in sub-Saharan Africa which are
severely affected by famine.**

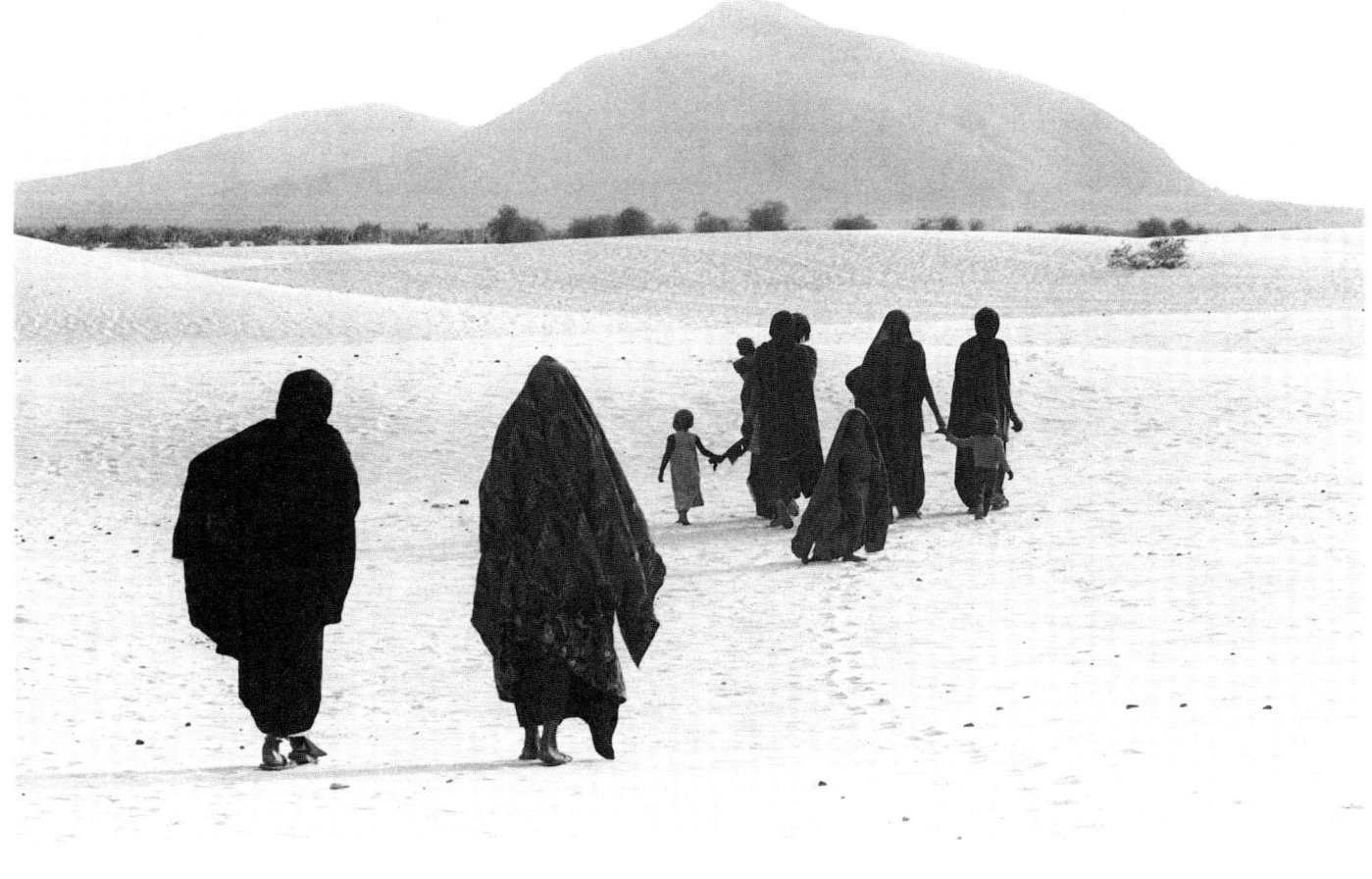

Seasonally on the move in search of grazing
for their animals, nomads camp in a dry
lake bed in northern Mali.

When pictures of the Ethiopian famine were shown on television in 1984, people throughout the industrialized world were shocked at the scale of human misery and the apparent hopelessness of the situation. Ordinary people dug into their pockets and sent money, while governments sent food and voluntary agencies sent skilled personnel, all in a desperate effort to contain the tragedy.

But the tragedy was not contained. In fact it has spread – to Sudan, Somalia, Chad, Mali and other countries of Africa's Sahel belt. Thirty million people in Africa are now affected by drought and famine, seven and a half million of them actually at risk of starving to death. This record level of world hunger has been reached despite the fact that at a global level there is enough food in the world to feed everybody.

Was the international aid just too little and too late? Or is something fundamentally wrong in Africa – something that makes life for many people so precarious that a sudden drought, or any other natural disaster, can tip the balance between survival and death? We should not be misled. It was not drought which caused the famine. Drought has merely served to accelerate a decline which is evident from Mali in West Africa to Ethiopia, thousands of miles away in the east. And in so doing, it has provided a tragic proof of the general failure of the policies of development. The millions of pounds spent have apparently not helped people to cope now that disaster has struck.

By April 1985, the public in Europe and America had donated several hundred million dollars to the small non-governmental organizations (NGOs) working to help the famine victims. The NGOs' emergency programmes have had extensive media coverage and gained widespread respect. But while airlifts of food or similar measures may succeed in bringing immediate relief, they can do nothing to remove the causes of distress.

Less attention has been paid to the more low-key, long-term development projects sponsored by the same non-governmental organizations. And yet if there have been any successes in development over the last decade, they are mainly to be found in the small, community-based projects to which the NGOs have turned. Few of the larger, government-controlled schemes have attempted to learn from their experience.

Over the last ten years the Sahelian countries, in West Africa, have received more aid per capita than anywhere else in the poor world. By contrast, rebel-held areas in Ethiopia have received relatively little assistance, because donors to these areas face charges by the Ethiopian government that they are financing revolt not development.

Looking at different approaches to development across sub-Saharan Africa, and at the processes whereby drought becomes disaster, we shall ask – is there an alternative to famine?

Introduction

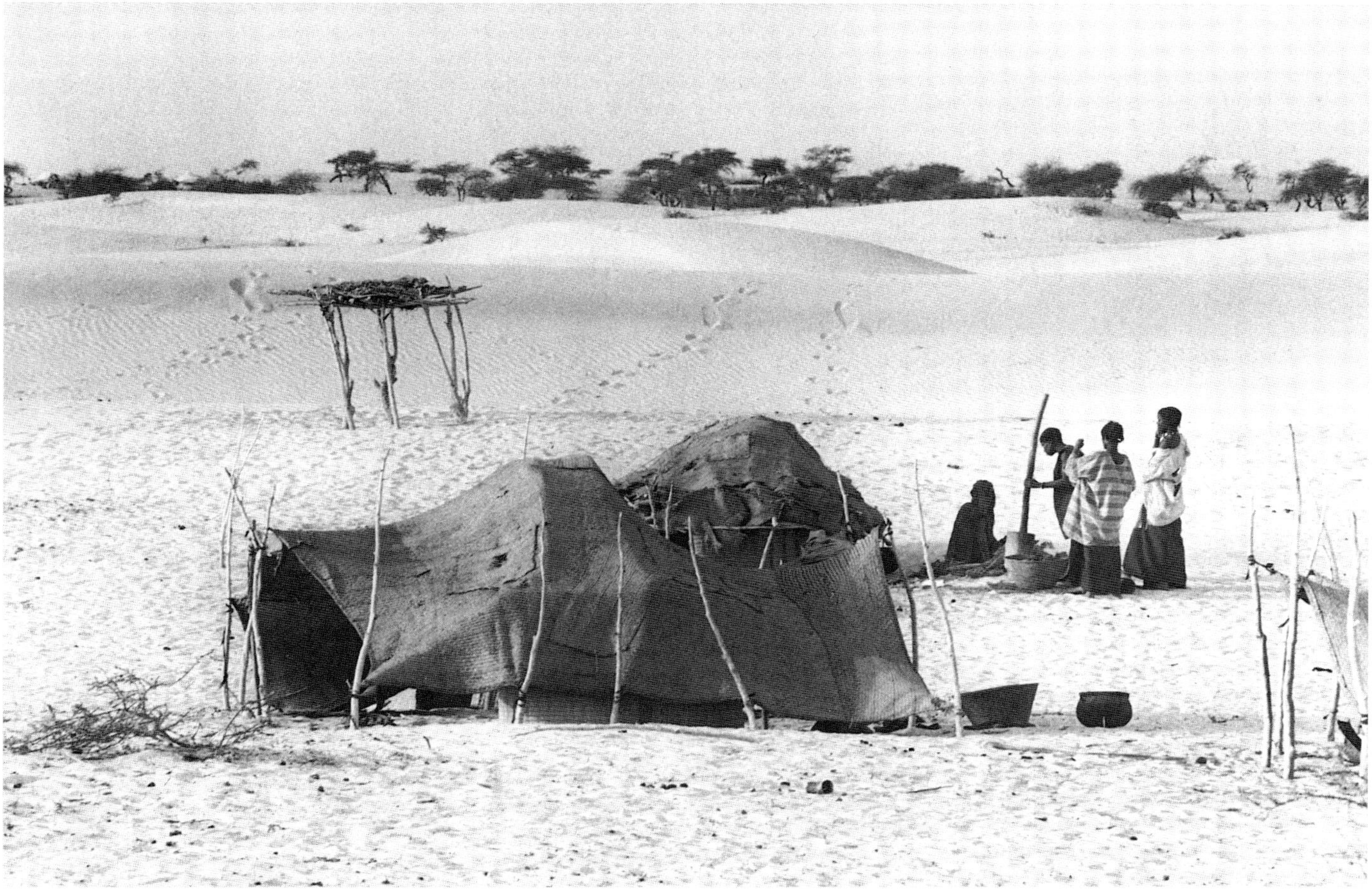

Over the ten years since the last famine, the Sahel countries of West Africa have received more aid money per person than anywhere else in the poor world. What difference has it made to the lives of these Malian nomads, now suffering from famine once again?

Aid goes to the developing world from western industrialized countries in the form of either grants or loans. 'Donors' does not therefore always accurately describe the relationship of the providers to the recipients of aid. The transfer of funds is effected in two main ways:

Bilateral aid is a direct arrangement between the governments of a rich and a poor country. The European countries and the United States have large bilateral aid programmes. Some funds take the form of grants, some of loans. Increasingly, the aid is linked to the purchase of goods and services from the donor country. For instance, a European government might give or lend the money to an African government for the construction of a power station or a paved road, providing that equipment, materials and skilled labour from the donor country were used in the project. This boosts the donor economy but does not necessarily give the recipient country what it most needs. Since 1980 it has been a requirement of British aid that it be linked to the British government's political and commercial interests.

Multilateral aid is the transfer of money to a poor country from a fund to which many countries contribute. There are many multi-lateral aid institutions, most but not all of which lend money to poor countries rather than give it to them. The loans may be 'soft' – interest-free or at a nominal rate of interest – or can be at rates up to normal commercial interest rates. Organizations lending money are, predictably, mainly attracted to large-scale potentially profitable projects rather than the needs of small farmers.

The International Monetary Fund (IMF) is the world's primary lending institution. Originally designed to meet the borrowing needs of industrialized countries, it now exercises a near monopoly in bailing out developing countries which face balance of payments problems. In recent years it has increasingly insisted that its monetarist prescriptions for economic reform are adopted by countries in receipt of its help.

The organizations of the United Nations (UN) are multilateral in structure. They both give grants and implement programmes. Much of their aid takes the form of technical assistance, the impact of which is fairly limited.

Between 1975 and 1980, $7.45 thousand million went to the Sahel in aid. About half of the money was in bilateral aid, and a quarter came through the multilateral agencies (excluding the OPEC and Arab development funds who provided about one fifth of the total). One fifth came from the UN.

The aid provided by charities, trusts and voluntary agencies is extremely small by comparison with the bilateral and multilateral donors. The former agencies – known collectively as non-governmental organizations (NGOs) – tend to concentrate on very small-scale projects and work directly with individual communities.

The donors

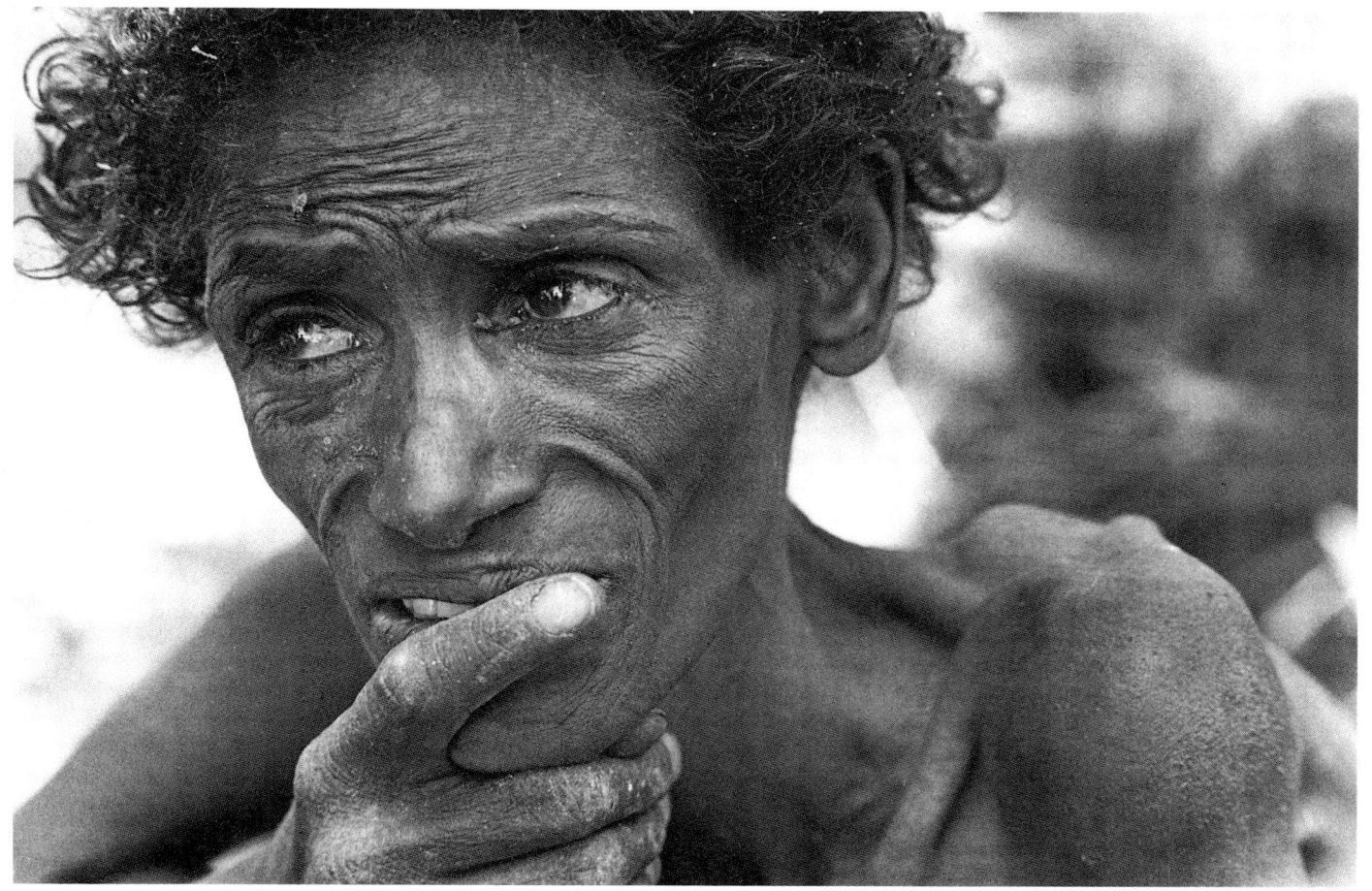

Tuberculosis was eradicated in the west 30 years ago. But because the treatment is long and expensive, contracting TB in the poor world is usually a death sentence. This woman is already ravaged by the disease.

THE SAHEL

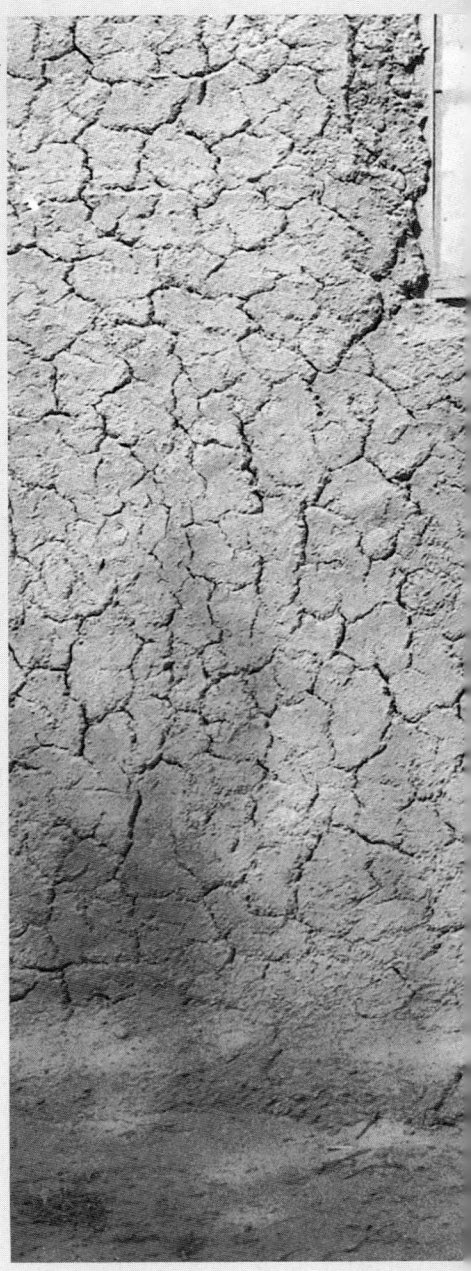

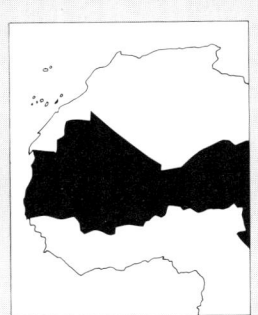

12

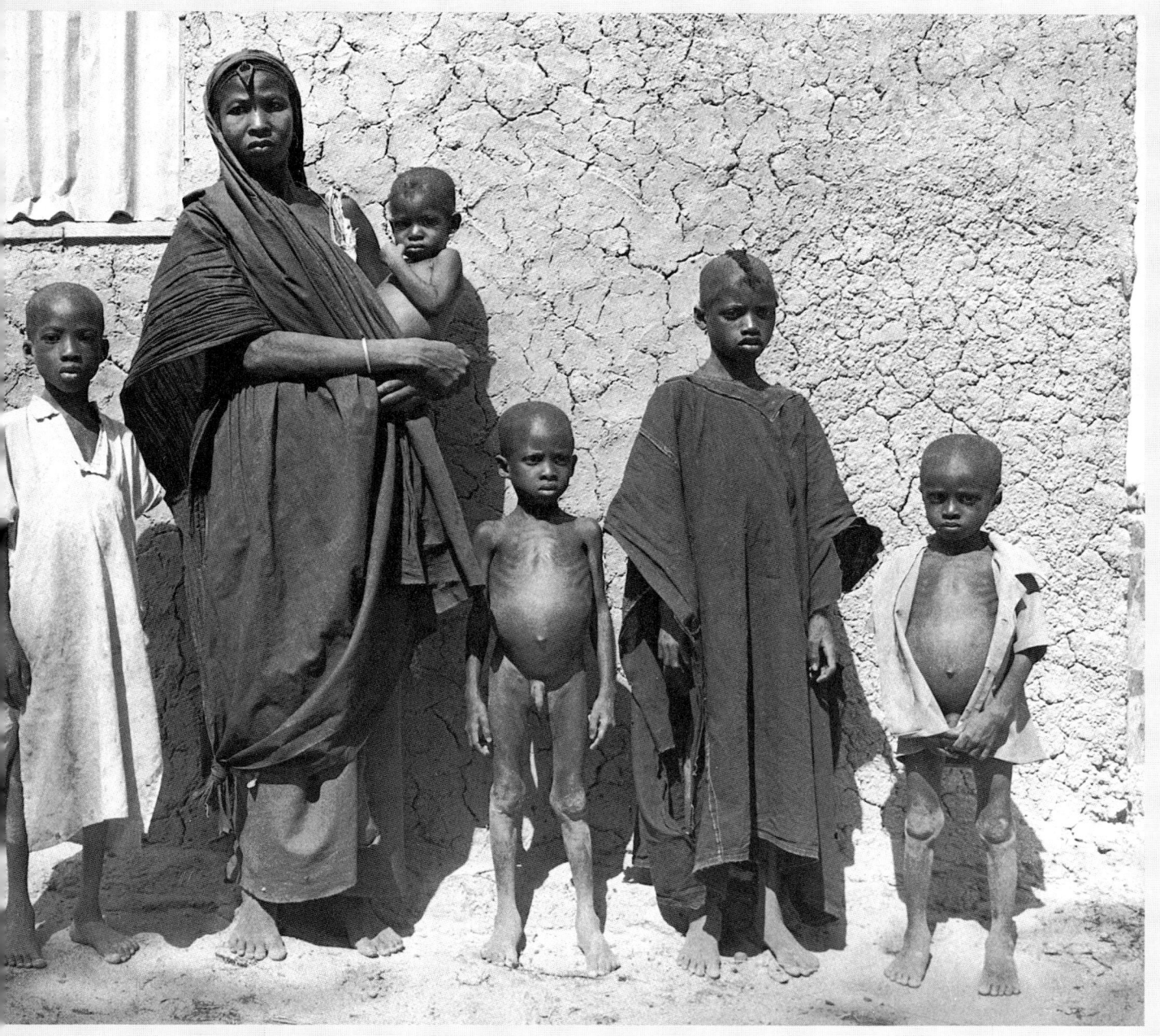

13

By December 1984, about 25,000 people were gathered in feeding camps around the ancient trading centre of Gao in Mali, 200 miles downstream from Timbuctoo on the river Niger. All were destitute. It was bitterly cold at night and few people had blankets. The cholera epidemic along the banks of the river had died down by then but measles was rampant. The cemetery was full and each day more bodies were being buried in the sand just outside the city.

All over the country poor peasant farmers and hungry nomads were leaving their homes in desperation, some after years of consecutive rain failure. But just 40 years ago, the French colonizers had dreams of using the vast irrigation potential in the flood plain of the river Niger to make Mali a breadbasket for Europe. In 1960, the country achieved independence, and it has since been the recipient of millions of dollars' worth of foreign aid. Why then are its people now unable even to feed themselves?

After the drought of the late 1960s, international development planners and the Malian government studied the national food production figures and concluded that the country's problem was one of overall lack of production. Their solution has been to attempt to increase that production, as fast as possible, on the assumption that if food is available then nobody will go hungry. Mali's fertile south has therefore been the target of most of the development programmes, with a view to encouraging this area to produce enough to feed the parts of the country where food production is more precarious.

This approach has not been restricted to Mali. It became the cornerstone of the World Bank's agenda for action in Africa, presented publicly in 1981 under the title 'Accelerated Development in sub-Saharan Africa'. The Bank's authors recommended 'targeting those areas where the physical resource base and existing human and physical infrastructure provide the pre-conditions for rapid payoff from additional investment'. In other words, they suggested working with more prosperous farmers who had already demonstrated their ability to grow more food than their neighbours or fellow countrymen. The resulting surplus, it was calculated, would quickly move countries towards food self-sufficiency.

Over the last ten years donors – including the United Nations and European and North American governments – have spent a thousand million dollars on development programmes. Most major agricultural projects have bypassed the poorest peasants and concentrated resources on 'pilot' entrepreneurial farmers in the more fertile parts of the country. Working with wealthier farmers is easier. They are better able to cope with debt since they have more collateral in the form of land and cattle, plus access to a bigger labour force. It is easier for state advisory services to make contact with fewer, larger farms than a large number of small ones. Farmers with a degree of financial security are also more able to take the risk of a new initiative, such as an unfamiliar seed type, whereas the very poor can scarcely afford to experiment with the family's food. These wealthier farmers are designated 'pilot farmers', and the thesis is that their poorer neighbours will gather round their fields, admire, and begin to imitate.

It is at this point that the theory fails in practice. Few neighbours do imitate. They have not received the training and are unlikely to be eligible for credit, nor do they have enough resources or land for innovations such as terracing or animal traction. In fact, the 'progress' being made by their neighbours may leave the poor in a worse position, through a number of unforeseen side effects. For instance, most farming in the Sahel is still done with a hand-held hoe, but increasing amounts of credit are being allocated for animal traction programmes.

One of the quickest ways for a farmer to produce a surplus with a plough is by persuading the village elders to allocate more land to him so he can generate a larger crop. Inevitably, the result is less land available to the rest of the villagers.

Most of Africa's own food production never reaches a market. It is grown by the family for the family. For development programmes to concentrate on increasing overall food availability in the market place (either through imports or through attempts to increase the surplus produced by successful farmers) is to misunderstand the nature of the problem facing the bulk of Africa's population.

Agriculture's successful response to market demand in the industrialized world has revolved around producing more food per acre using less people. The trend has been towards larger farms employing a smaller labour force, with increasing use of mechanization and manufactured fertilizers. Most development models promoted in sub-Saharan Africa have reflected this approach. Higher yields have been produced through the use of hybrid seeds, fertilizer and pesticide – highly questionable policy in a continent where money is in short supply but labour is abundant.

World Bank strategy has not been limited to encouraging key producers with aid packages. Towards the end of 1981, several western governments' aid missions in Mali, led by the Bank, decided that the Malian state bureaucracy was the main hindrance to increased production. In particular, they cited state control of the grain market and the low price being offered to farmers for their food crops as disincentives to production. Threatened with aid cutbacks from these donors, the Malian government agreed to a policy of what became known as 'liberalization'. But, although in theory the state had a monopoly on all cereals bought and sold in the country, in reality its share

14

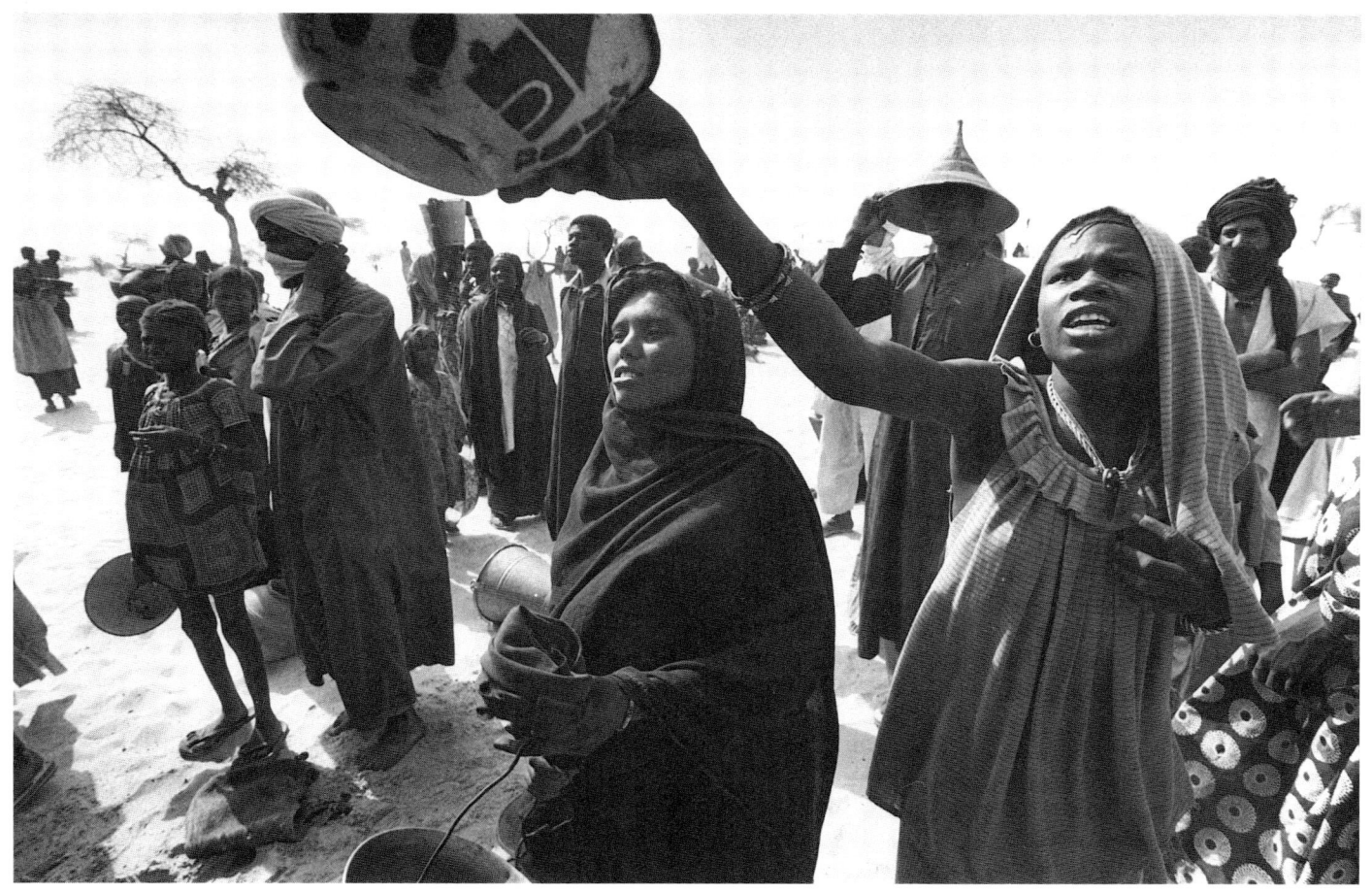

In many parts of Mali there is an acute
shortage of water; drought has left wells
depleted or empty. Here, a European aid
agency brings water for a few people by
tanker from Goundam, a town five hours'
drive away.

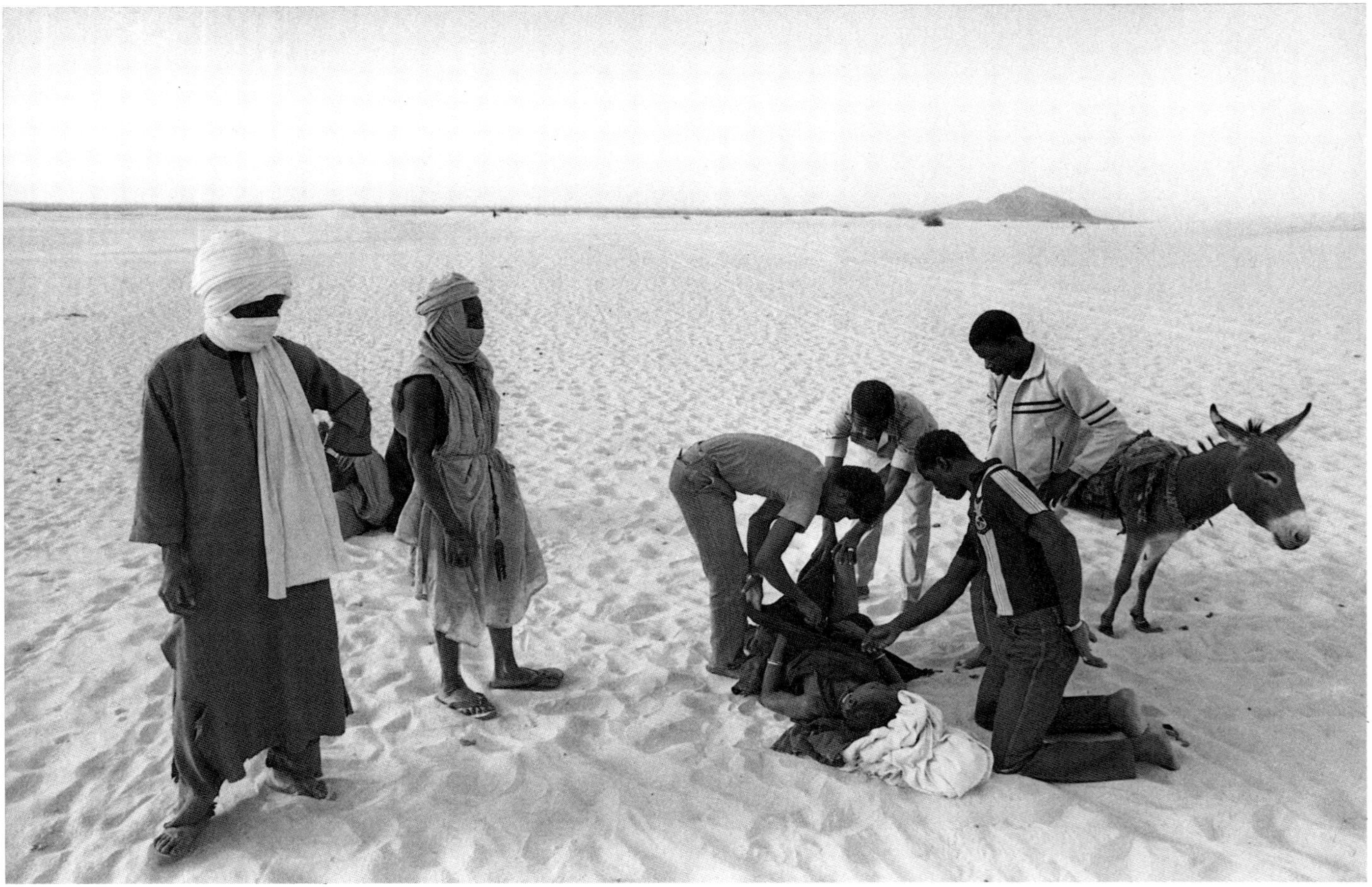

In Mali in late 1984, an epidemic of cholera
began to spread through a nomad
population already weakened by drought.
Hundreds of people died before a
European relief agency helped to contain
the outbreak.

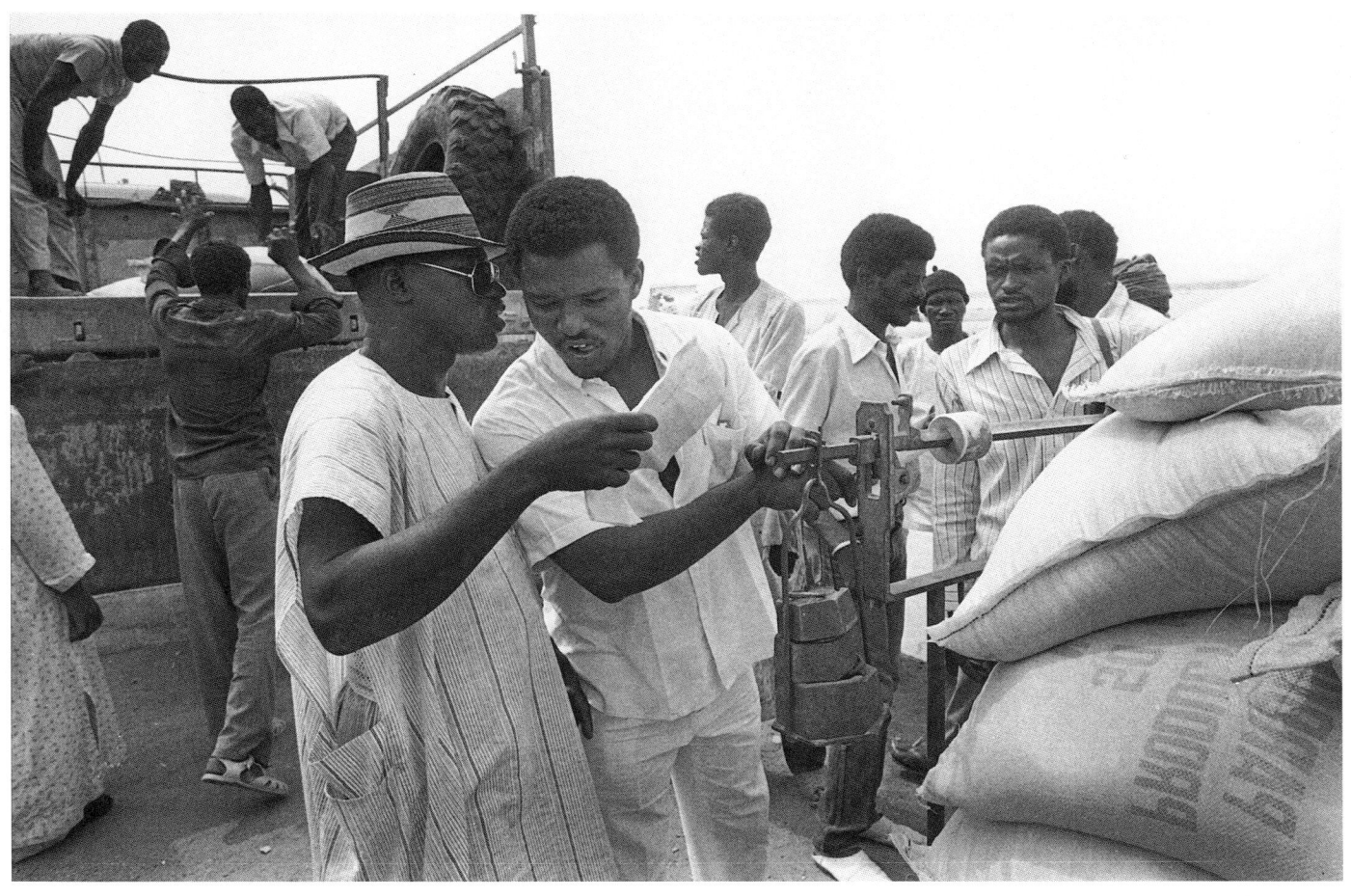

Merchants co-operate with each other to raise the going price for grain. In times of shortage, it becomes impossible for the poor to meet the cost of staple foods.

was less than 20 per cent. Nonetheless, that supposed monopoly was abolished and the state's already small share of the market decreased. At the same time it was agreed that the state should pay more for its grain, on the premise that if the private traders followed suit then the overall increase in purchase prices should encourage farmers to grow additional food which they could sell.

Malian traders immediately took advantage of their new-found liberty. Now, wherever grain is to be bought, they buy it. Wherever there is market demand they are happy to supply it. 1985 is a good example. The 1984 harvest deficit was around 400,000 tonnes because of the drought, but by December the four major private traders had already brought 300,000 tonnes of additional grain into the country, for sale to anybody with the money to pay for it.

There is no evidence so far of increased production, only of increased activity, by fewer people, in the market place. When most people have no spending power a free market place does not solve their problems. Some argue that the combination of singling out successful farmers and opening up the market place has made the lives of the poor even more difficult. In the current tragedy, aid planners have little choice but to accept that few of the millions of dollars spent have benefitted those who most needed assistance. One senior American aid planner put it very bluntly when he said, 'The damn thing hasn't worked'.

18

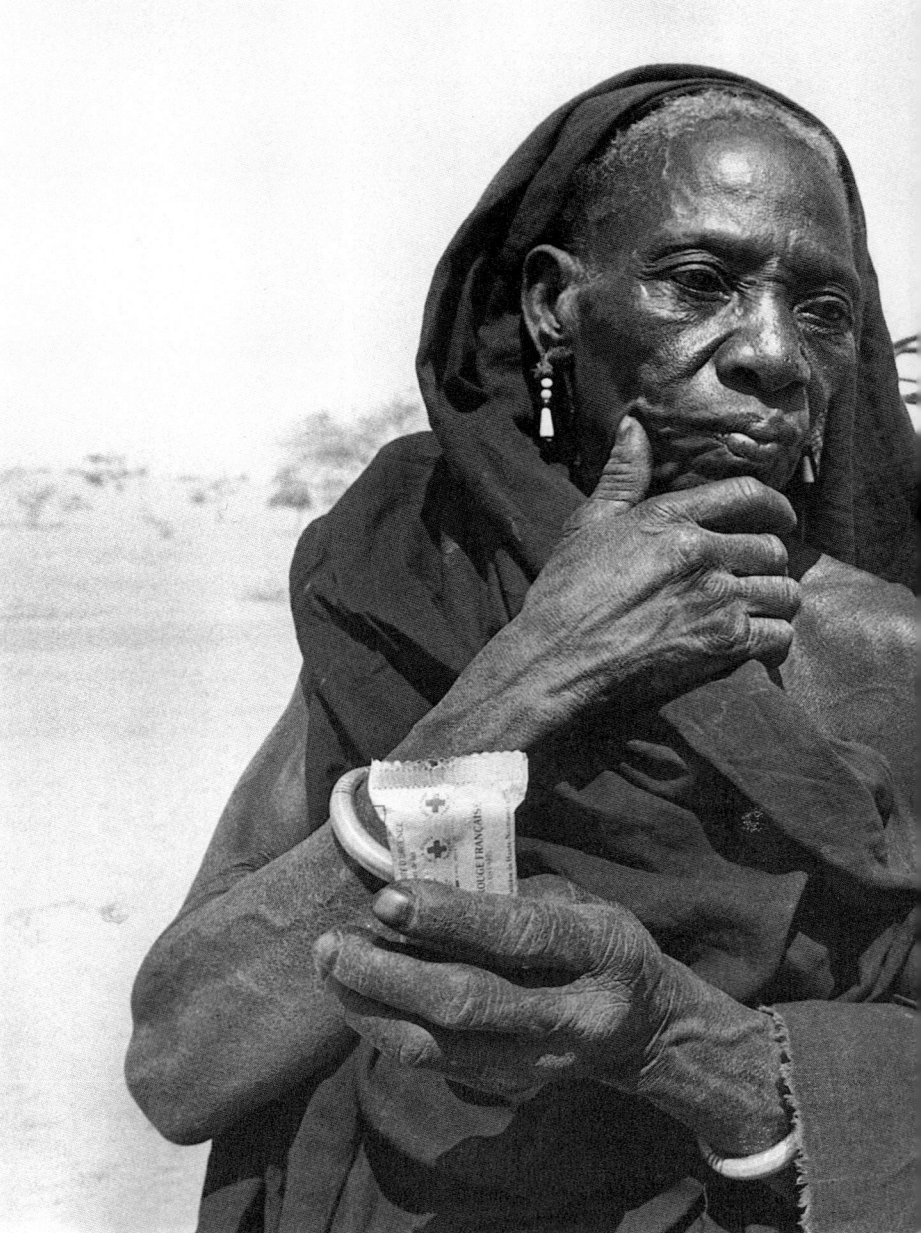

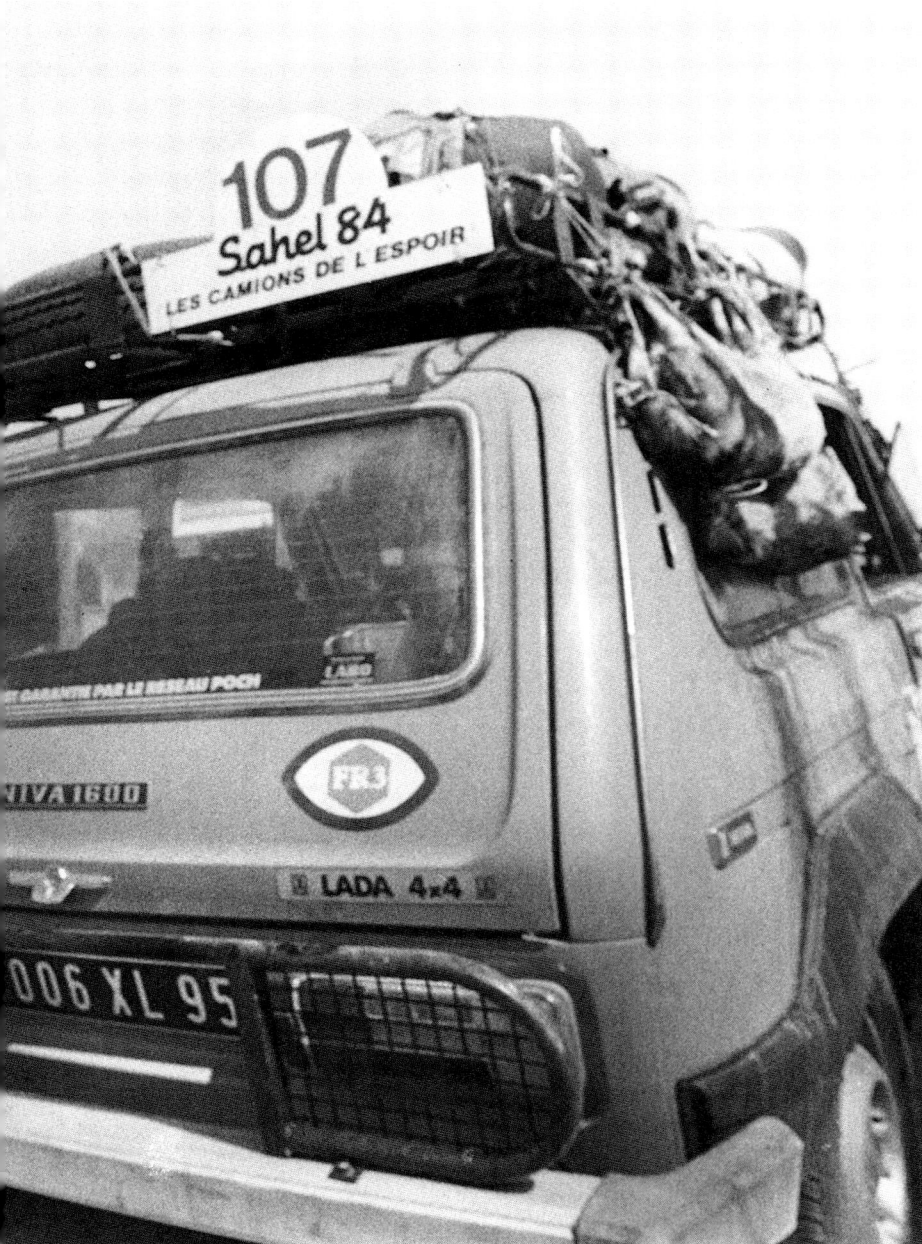

A French truck rally, 'Les Camions de l'Espoir', on a mercy mission across the Sahel desert from Senegal to Niger, for which the French public donated 40 million francs. The 'Trucks of Hope' turned into a strange carnival, as the convoy, accompanied by 30 journalists, two TV crews and two light aircraft, raced across the desert distributing 12,000 cases of individually-wrapped, high-protein biscuits, medical supplies and agricultural equipment. The execution of the project was so ill-considered that one of the truck drivers was prompted to remark, 'We have raised money from the poor of the rich countries to give to the rich of the poor countries'.

19

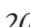

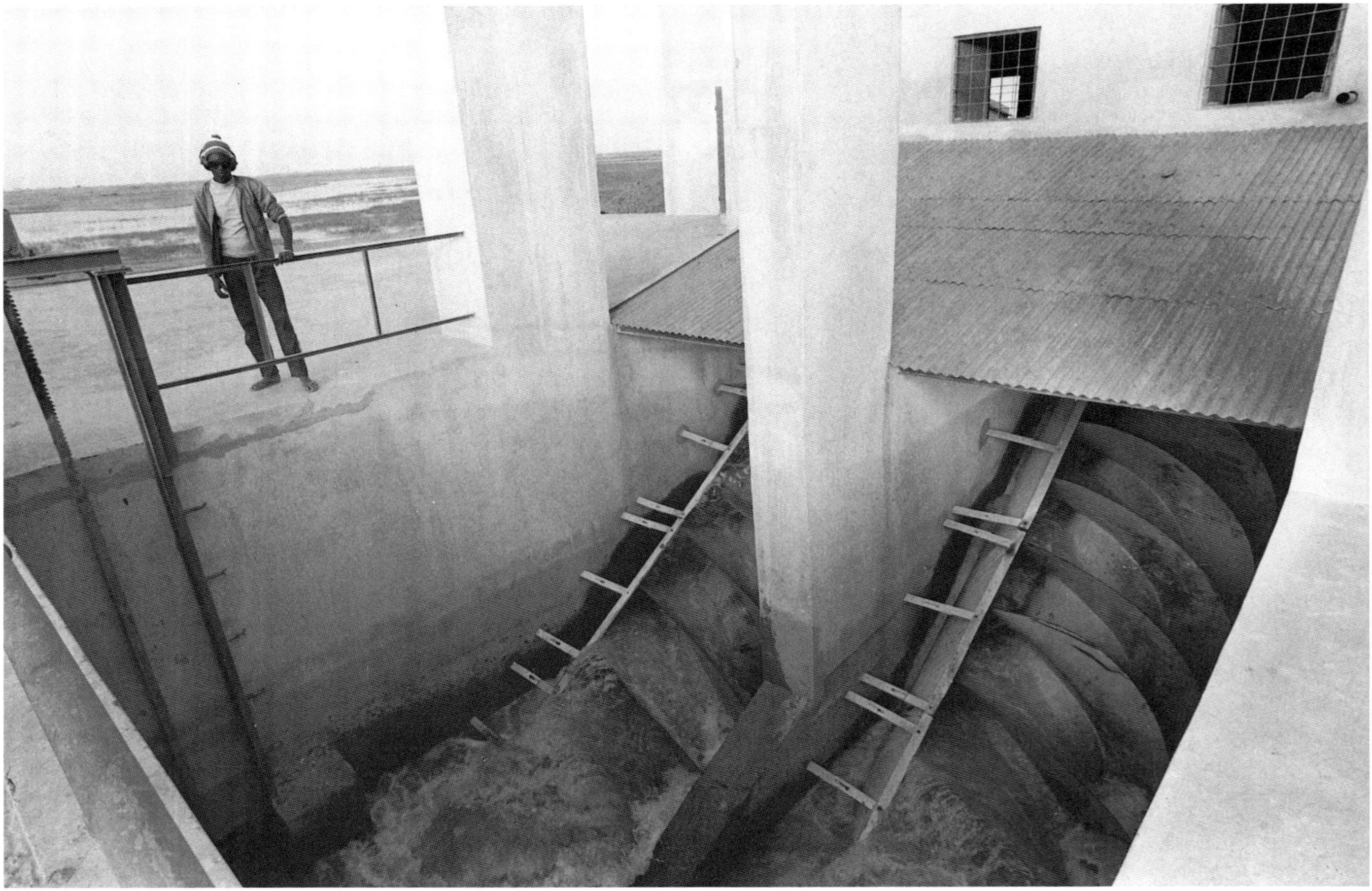

Many development projects are characterized by lack of foresight. This project near Timbuctoo in Mali is designed to irrigate 1,000 acres, using diesel-driven Archimedes screws to lift water out of the River Niger. When the river floods late and to a low level, the project's design means that water cannot reach the bottom of the screws until late in the growing season. The farmers' rice harvests are poor as a result, but they still have to pay for the fuel and fertilizer.

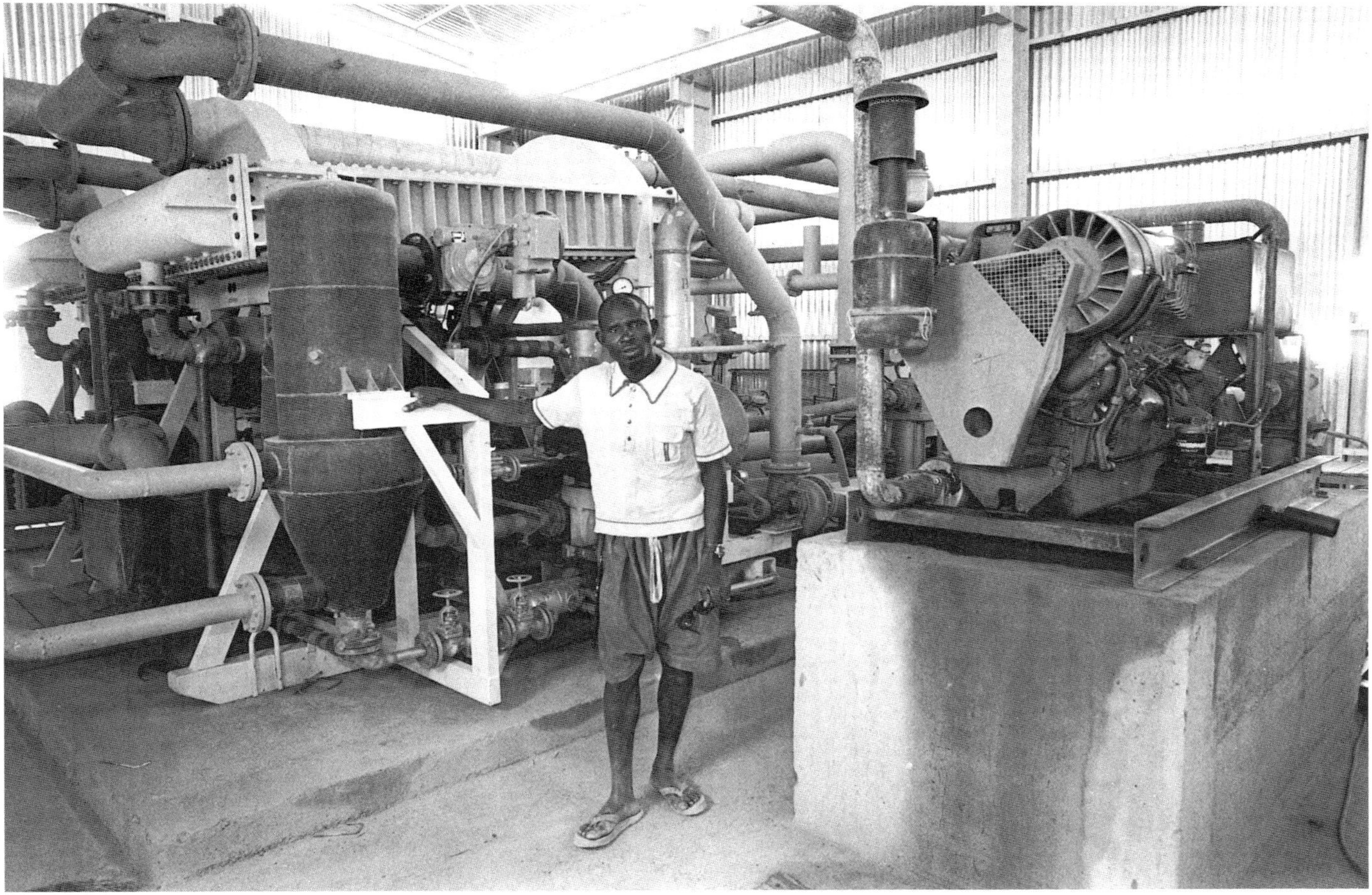

This solar energy irrigation project at Diré in Mali cost $1 million, and was built with bilateral aid from a European government. Its complex design, together with insufficient provision for maintenance, meant that when it failed after working for 200 hours, it never ran again. A standby diesel motor (right) now pumps the irrigation water.

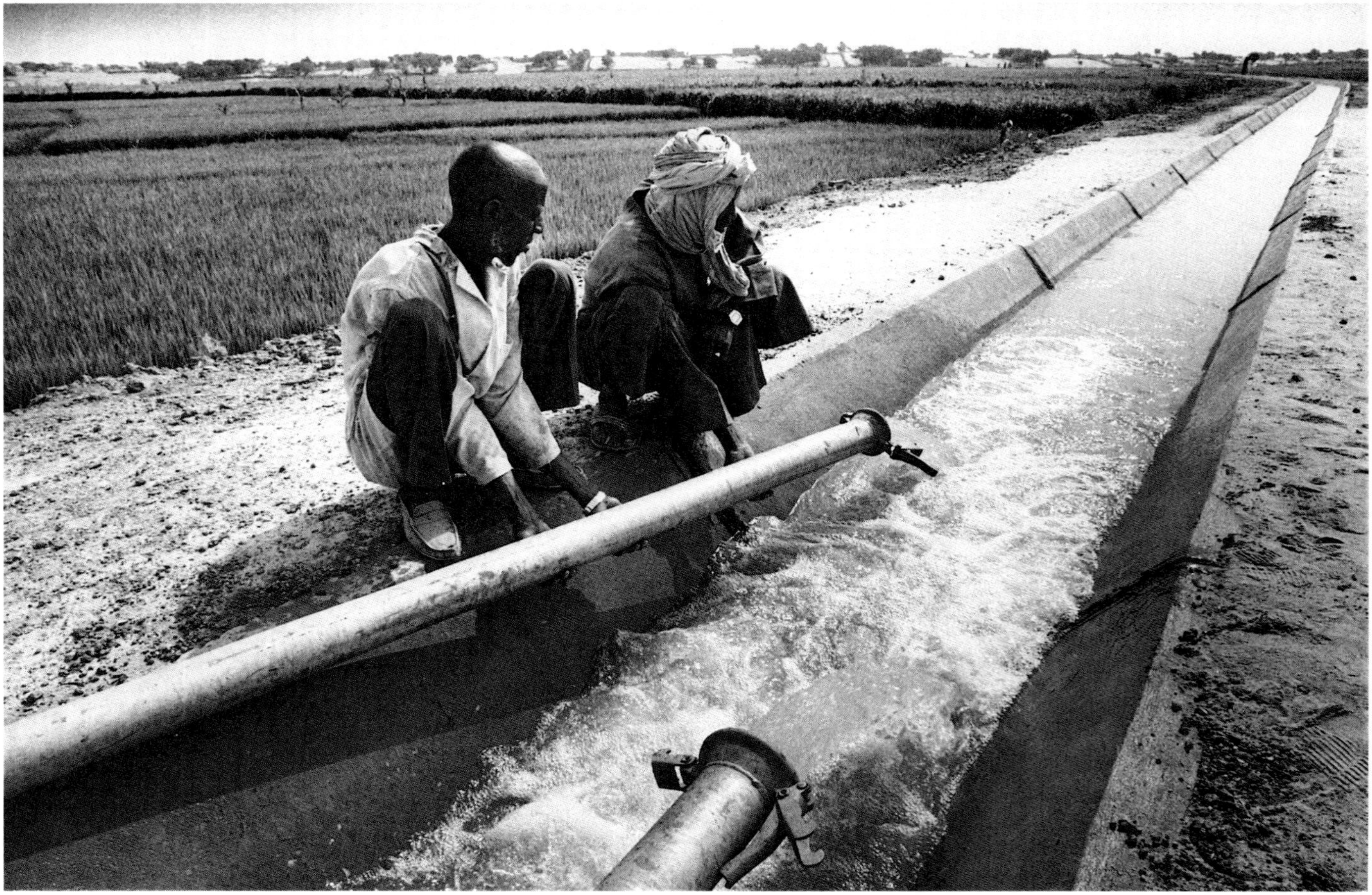

Some development programmes are culturally inappropriate. Here, Malian peasants provide the labour on an irrigation scheme near Gao which produces three harvests a year. The method demands continual intensive labour; this system is not well suited to the lifestyle of subsistence farmers, which traditionally revolves around community and family affairs as well as farming.

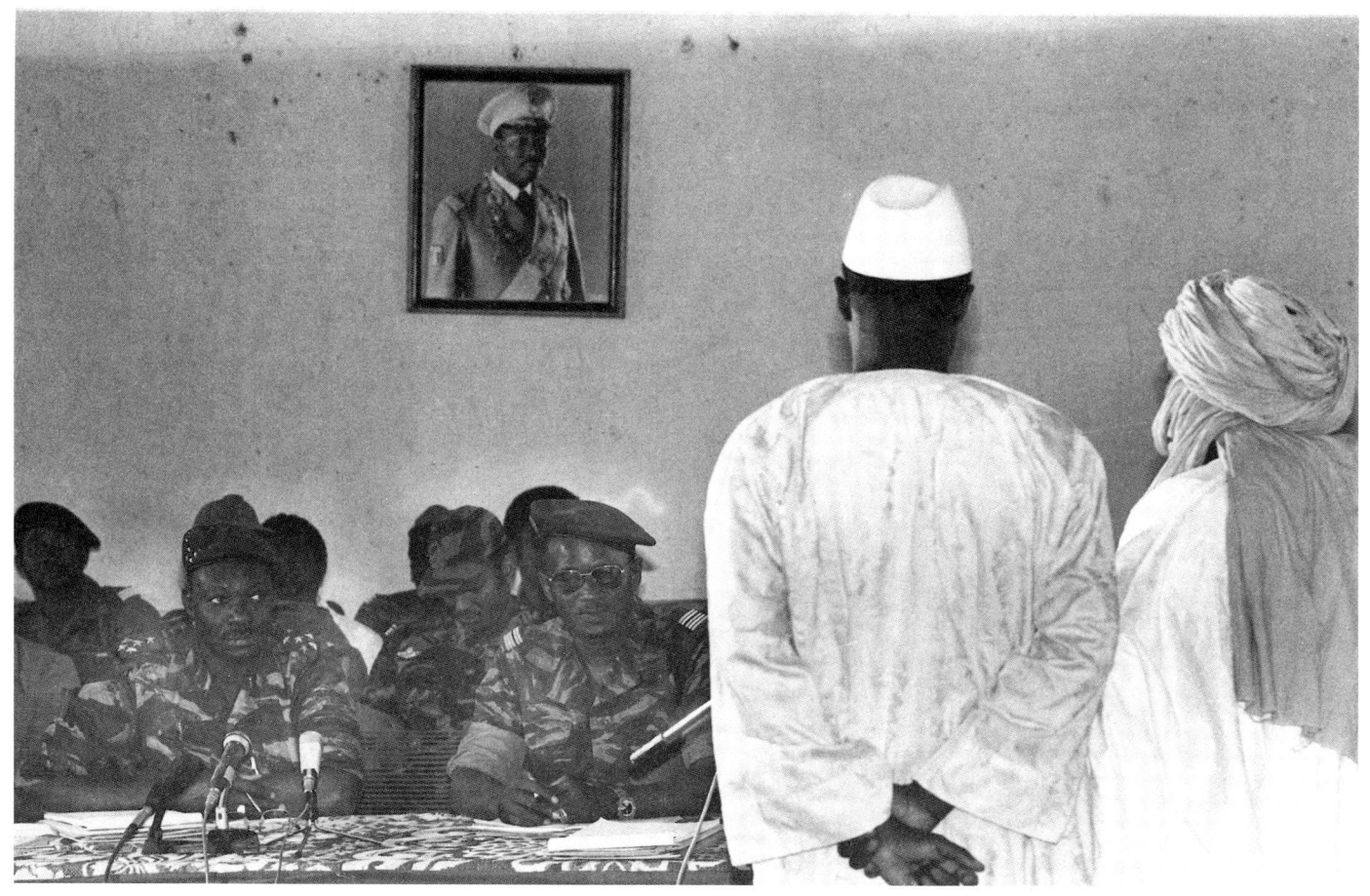

Dissatisfaction with the economic policies imposed by the World Bank is increasing amongst the population in Mali. General Traore, President of Mali, (left, and in the portrait above), visits community leaders in Diré to hear their views on current agricultural developments in the area.

Credit for the production of cash crops for export is an important programme in the Sahel. During the colonial period, groundnuts were the primary source of profit for the European cooking oil industry. Now their overcultivation has almost destroyed the soil in the northern part of Senegal. We can watch the same process at work with cotton production in Burkina Faso. Cotton only occupies four per cent of cultivated land at present, but its production exercises a near monopoly on the agricultural advice and resources provided by the state for the more fertile parts of the country. Seeds, fertilizers and pesticides for cotton production are provided on credit by the state to those with the necessary collateral. The loan is then repayable at harvest time.

Cotton farmers have a guaranteed market. After the harvest, the state-owned cotton company's lorries arrive to take away the crop. One farmer in south west Burkina Faso explained that 'when we grow cotton we know what we will be paid. Next year, we will grow more cotton and less millet'. Not surprisingly, cotton production has increased more than 30 times since independence in 1960, while food production has stagnated. For those farmers with the resources to choose what to grow, food crops have been financially less attractive.

Continuous cultivation of cotton is slowly destroying the Sahelian soil. Africa has less young and rich soils than any other continent, and the weathered sandy surface of the Sahel lacks many important elements. Traditionally, land was rotated between crops, or at least left fallow to enable the soil and vegetative cover to regenerate after cultivation. But farmers who take credit have to repay it through intensive use of the land. There is now very little left fallow in the cotton-producing areas of the country.

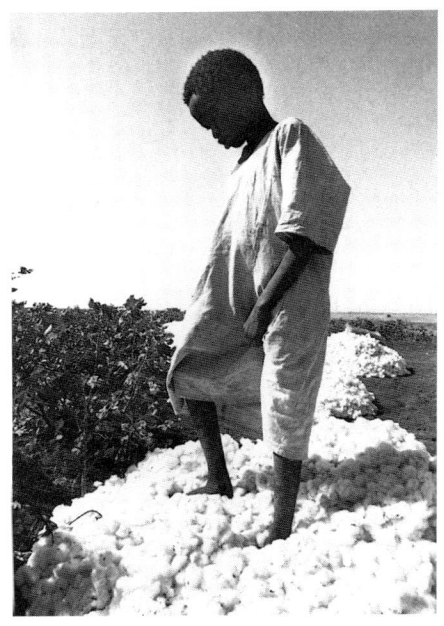

Cotton awaiting collection by truck.

Cotton requires more pesticides than almost any other crop. The continuous use of cotton fertilizer, without the complementary addition of organic matter such as compost, is slowly acidifying the soil and reducing its fertility. The same fertilizer is widely used on cereal crops, although not well adapted to them, since it is the only fertilizer available in much of the country. Its destructive effects are therefore not limited to the cotton-growing areas.

Despite this ecological damage, cotton is a crop which is much encouraged in the Sahel by both Sahelian governments and their donors. Food production in drought- and war-stricken Chad has collapsed, but the country has nonetheless increased its cotton yields to become the second largest producer in Africa. In Mali, one American aid project designed to increase food production is insisting that all farmers who take credit from the project give over part of their land to cotton, which effectively becomes the scheme's collateral. The Americans aim to provide credit to the entire community, with the implication that everybody will sacrifice some food production for the export crop.

Credit for cotton production is offered to men, without taking into account the effect on the other half of the population. Although women have traditionally been important and independent growers of food, with their own land and rights over the harvest, they

24

Impact of cash cropping

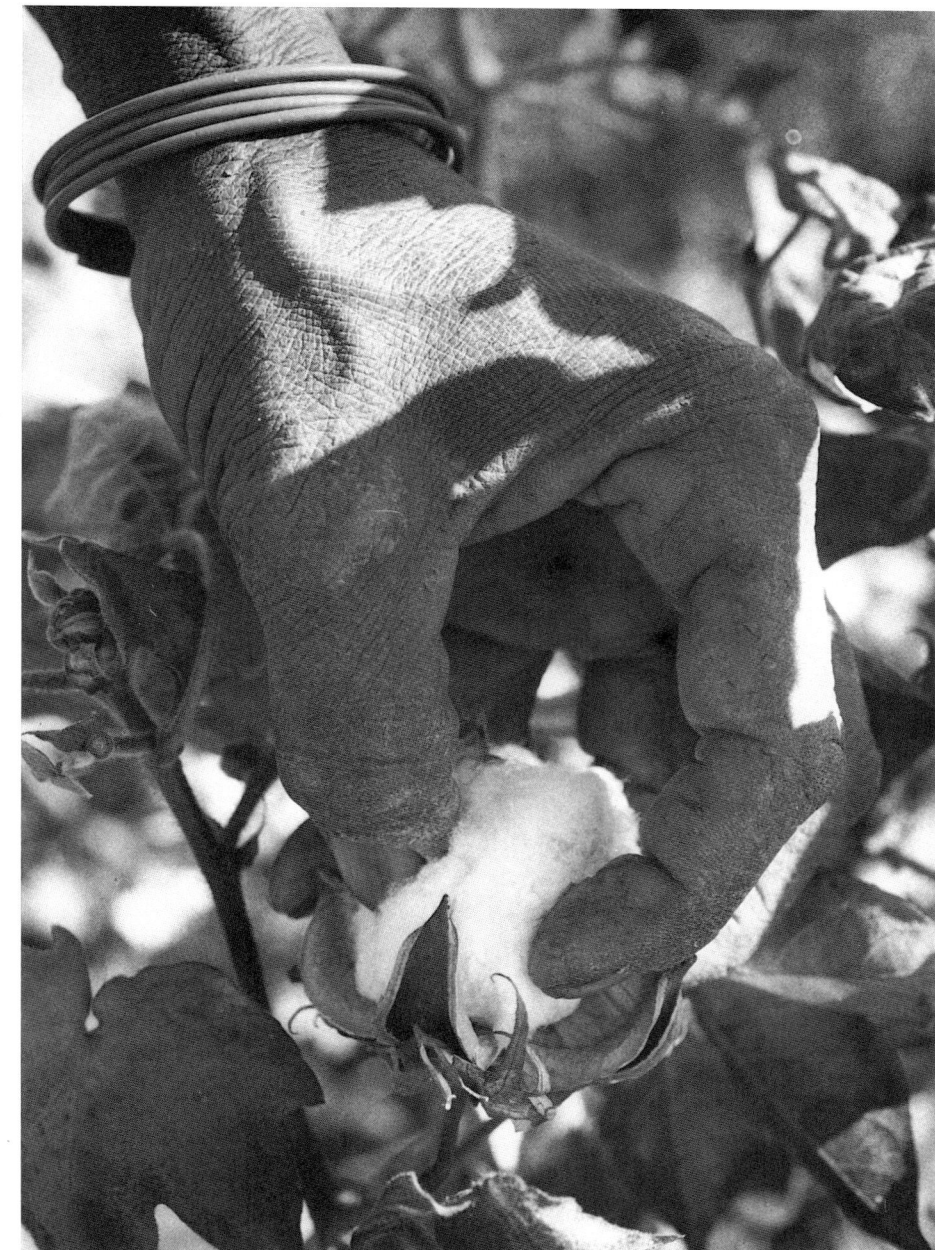

Cotton harvesting.

are simply used as labourers in cotton production. They have less time and energy to devote to their own essential food crops, and few rights over any profit their husbands may make on the cotton crop.

Inappropriate to the poor

Most of the Sahel's people are subsistence farmers, scratching out next year's food from the soil. If their harvest fails they do not have the capital to buy food on the open market, particularly at the high prices charged by private traders. They are unable to participate in many of the aid schemes, and the technical packages which suit a wealthy farmer are simply not applicable to the poor peasant with minimal means of production.

Floating rice fails after poor rains.

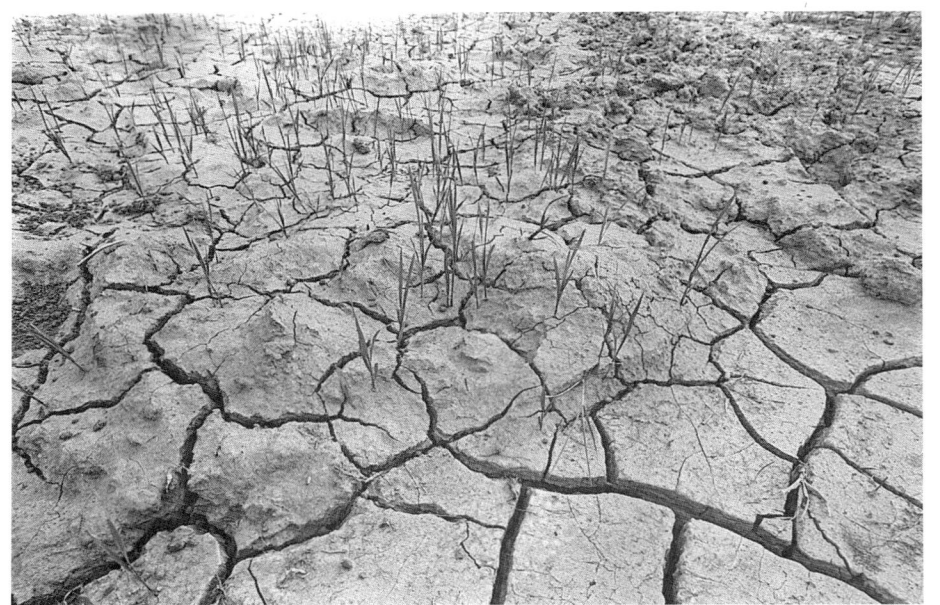

If the family's survival depends on the food they manage to coax out of their small patch of near-arid land, they need to be extremely sure of new techniques before risking experiments. This hesitation can result in their exclusion from a programme. A group of local co-operatives working on agricultural improvement schemes in northern Ghana limited their size to 150 members. The poorest people in the community watched very carefully to see whether the new initiative was going to be worth the precious investment of labour and the annual membership fee. By the time they had decided that it was a worthwhile programme, it was too late, and membership had already closed.

One reason for the apparent bias towards programmes which benefit richer farmers is that it is much harder for aid planners to devise agricultural programmes which are appropriate to the poor. Until the aid planners talk to the real 'experts', the poverty-stricken peasants in whose name the programmes are undertaken, aid is likely to continue to fail.

As well as needing access to capital and the land to grow food, any farmer requires a labour force. This is one resource over which the Sahel's poor have some control. One reason for having large families is to enable people to work their land even harder, or to extend over more land, whatever the quality. But for families to cultivate so intensively is often to dig their own grave. The soil becomes progressively more infertile and eventually incapable of feeding everybody who depends on it. It is only then that a 'population problem' is identified, only then that the rural poor are seen as a burden on the state and the international community. But high population figures do not necessarily result in mass hunger. Part of the blame must be laid at the door of western development models which use mechanization and artificial fertilizer in preference to human energy. These development techniques might eventually raise the food production statistics of the Sahel, and help to feed the townspeople, but they will be irrelevant, and possibly harmful, to the millions of subsistence farmers who are increasingly failing to grow their own food and who lack the capital to buy somebody else's surplus.

One farmer in northern Burkina Faso explained very clearly how he used to farm a plot of land with his father. The size of the family grew but the harvest did not. Lacking the cash to buy fertilizers, they over-cultivated the land in an effort to produce more food. That land is now exhausted and the farmer has no options open to him. He is too poor to buy animals which could manure his fields, has no capital to invest in fertilizers and has no time to leave the land fallow. He fully expects that he will have to abandon the plot he cultivates with his sons.

26

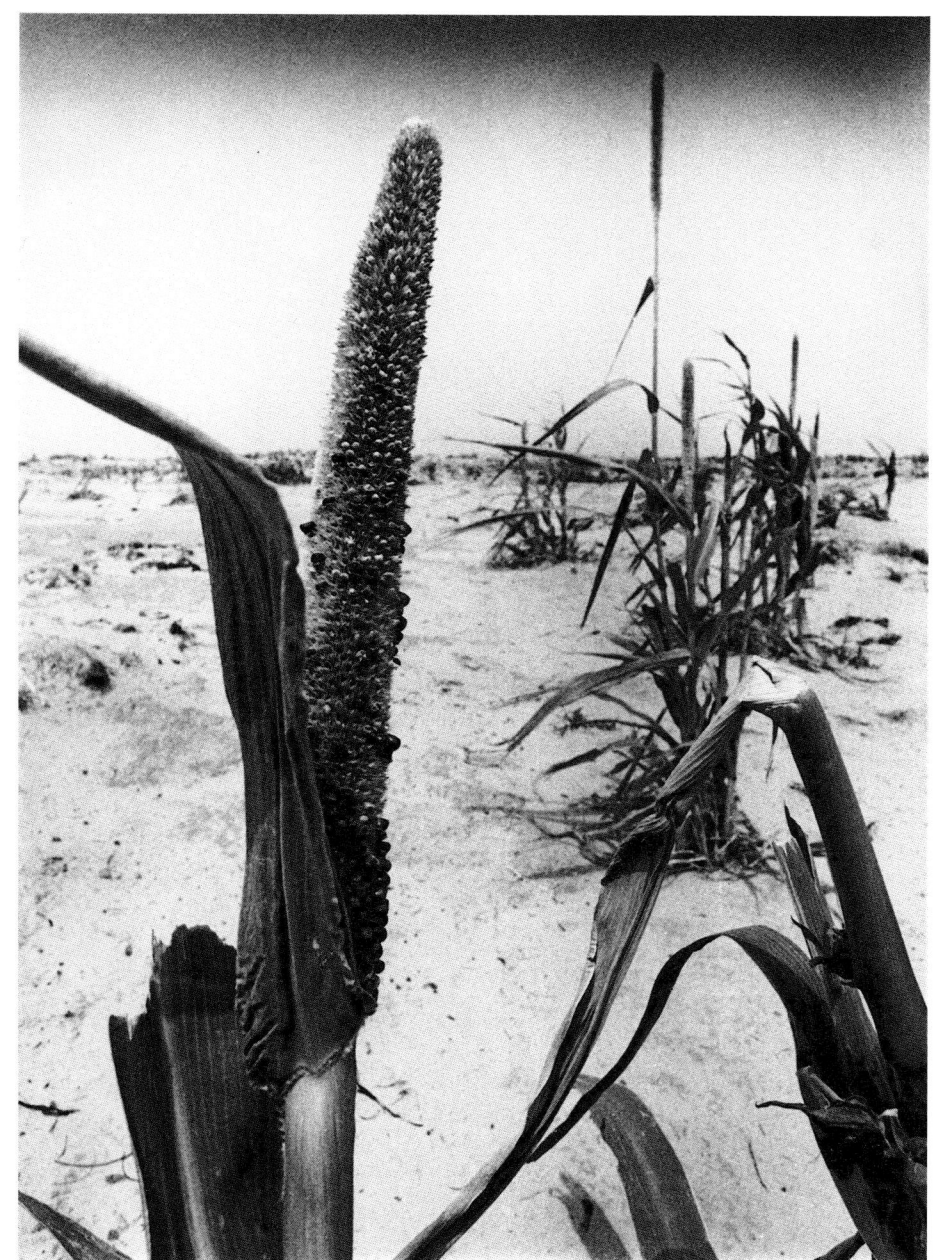

A failed millet crop grown on semi-desert land by poor farmers. The land is better suited to pasture for nomads' animals than farmers' crops.

The popular image of the desert taking over farmland at a speed of several miles a year is inaccurate. The spread of the desert is more like a bad skin disease. Outbreaks appear wherever people have exhausted their land by overworking it. The individual patches then join together, leading to the day when the entire body will be affected.

Falling harvests compounded by drought have led the Sahel's poor to attempt to farm ever more marginal land, usually close to the edge of the desert. This land is marginal because of the minimal and unpredictable rainfall it receives. Despite the farmers' efforts, it remains largely unsuitable for cultivation. In many parts of the Sahel, life can only be sustained through the flexible nomadic form of society, in which herdsmen track down the pockets of good pasture created by localized showers. There are five million pastoralists (cattle-herders) spread throughout large areas of land in the Sahel, and pursuing a way of life developed in direct response to poor and upredictable patterns of rainfall.

Traditionally, the pastoralists combine their skill at seeking out available pasture with spreading their stock thinly over large areas. This ensures that no area is over-grazed. Some groups in the Sahel practise true nomadism, moving more or less continuously and following no set pattern. Others move their livestock along pre-determined routes each year. During the dry season, herd numbers are effectively limited by the amount of pasture within reach of the animals' base well. Other grazing is provided at this time of year by the harvested fields of farmers, where the cattle graze the stubble, manure the ground, and then move on before the farmer needs the land again for sowing. Some cattle stay and graze on fallow land, but when the rains begin the Sahel's grasses start to grow again and most nomads move their animals away from the wells, allowing the surrounding pasture to recover before the next dry season.

In any one year, poor rainfall can result in reduced vegetation, which the herdsmen traditionally cope with through local migration or through the sale of surplus stock. In subsequent years of good rainfall, they regain their economic position. These cyclical patterns of good and bad years of rainfall are the norm with which the pastoralists have always lived. But they have always led a separate life, not well integrated with their national governments which operate from offices in faraway towns. Their needs have been understood neither by their governments nor by western 'experts', and their traditional systems have been weakened by many agricultural developments. Intensified farming is steadily whittling away fallow land and destroying a critical part of the ecological base on which their survival depends. One of the most damaging trends has been the spread of settled farming

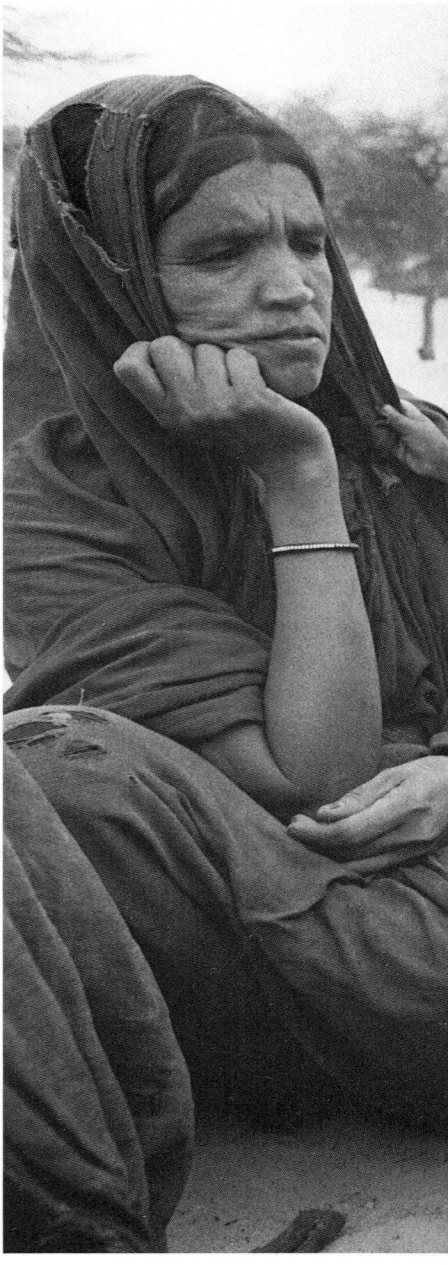

28

The spreading desert

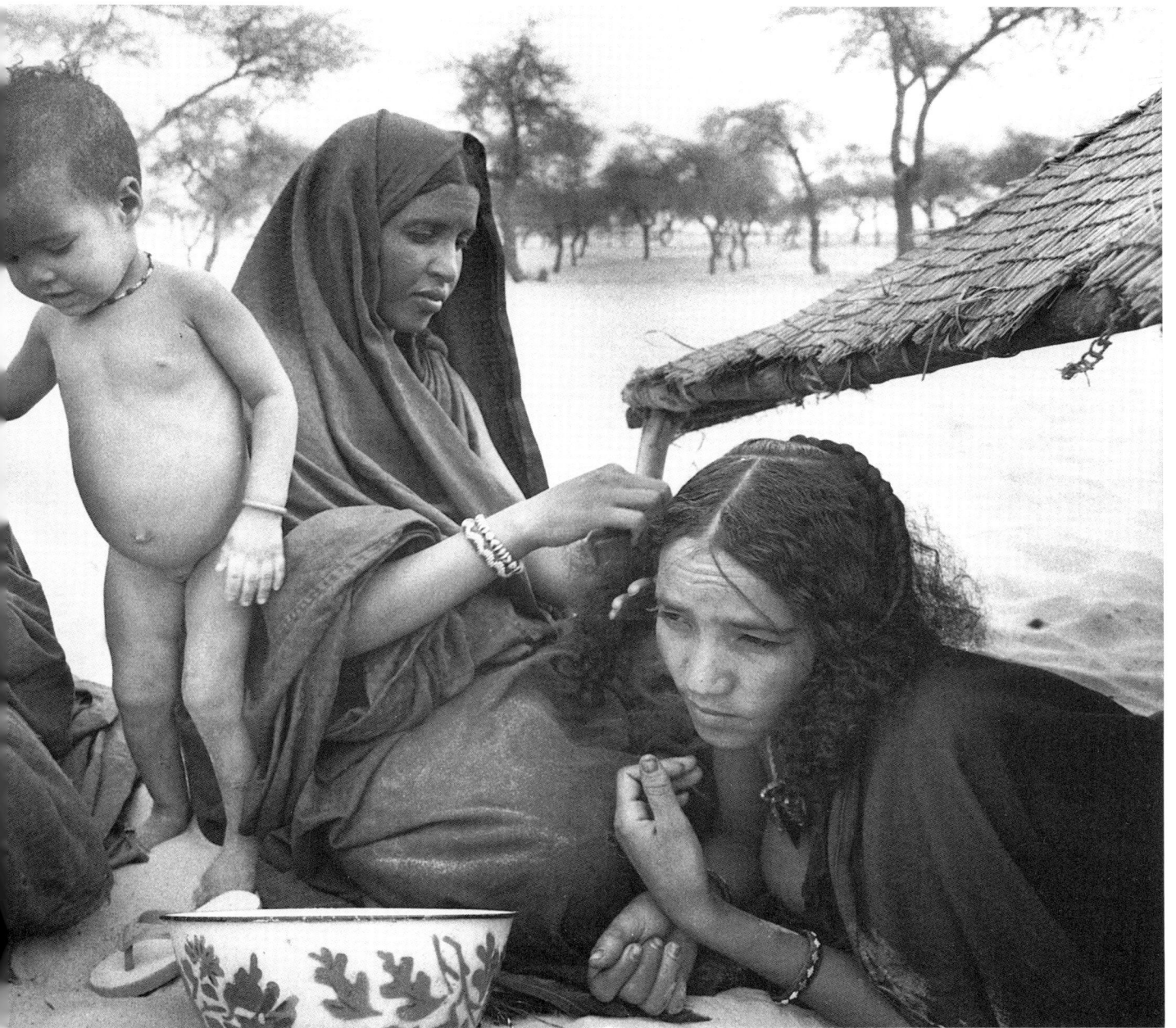

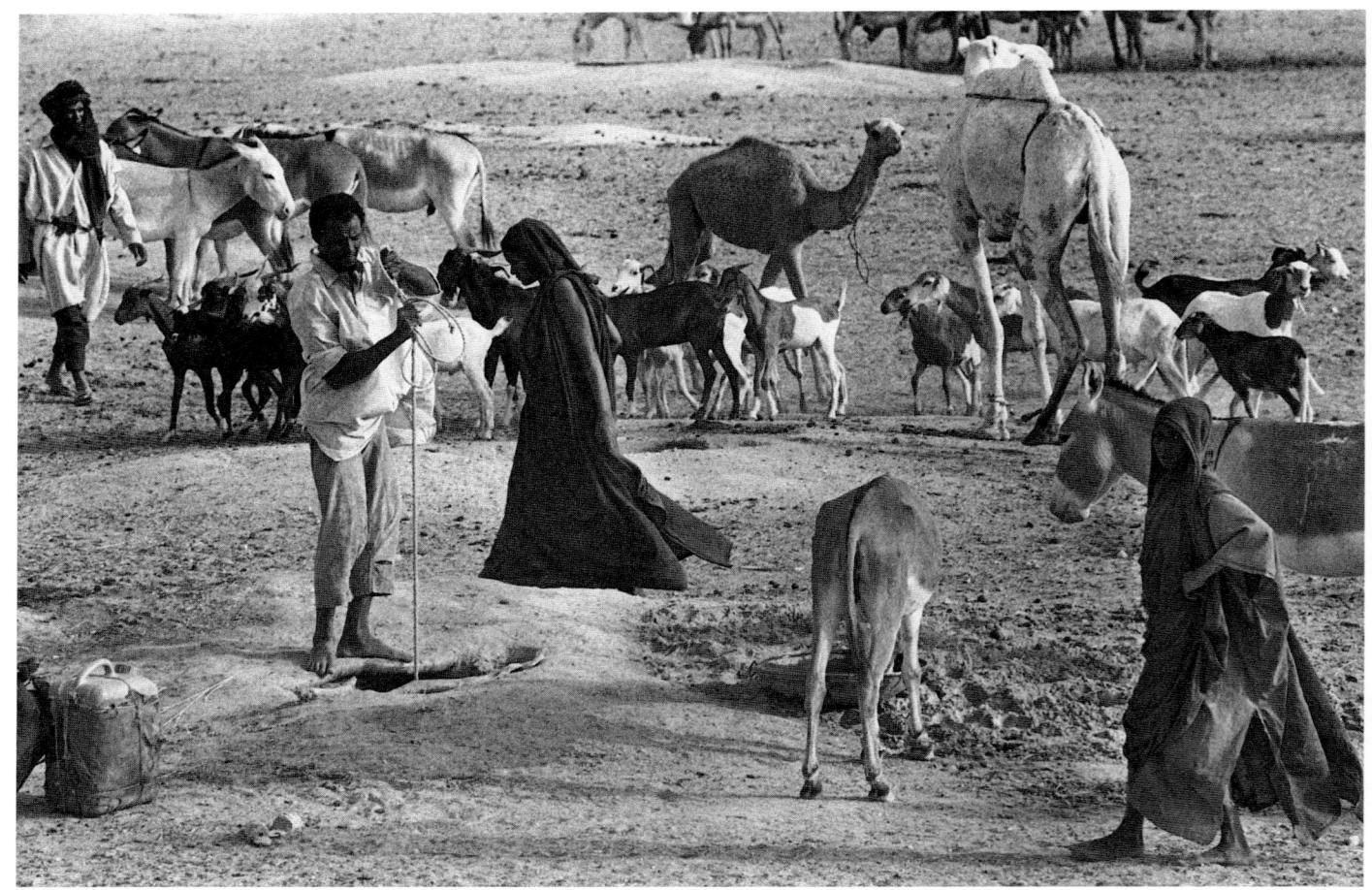

Many shallow wells and water holes have disappeared in the drought. Since animals can only travel a limited distance from their water source, the amount of pasture land available to them has been further reduced by the drought.

Previous page: Some Tuaregs have had to abandon their nomadic lifestyle and have gathered around the towns. This family, camped near Timbuctoo, now survives by selling Tuareg souvenirs and camel rides to tourists.

The Tuaregs' economy depends on animals which they keep for milk or trade for grain. As pasture land decreases, malnutrition increases among the nomads.

into the traditional grazing lands of the pastoralists.

Throughout the Sahel, the poorest peasants have exhausted their land and been forced on to the 'marginal' areas they previously left unused. In doing so, they have squeezed the pastoralists, dependent on access to large areas of land, on to ever smaller areas. Increasing restrictions on their movements by farmers desperate for a harvest are resulting in ecological disaster.

Those aid programmes which have directed themselves towards the Sahelian nomads have in the main perceived the problem of shortage of drinking water for the herds, but have failed to recognize the corresponding grazing needs. Since the 1950s, European government aid has established a network of deep boreholes with pumps to replace the much larger number of (albeit unreliable) traditional shallow wells. But these new wells effectively *diminished* the amount of pasture available, since cattle can only travel a limited distance from their water supply to graze. It was hoped that the new boreholes would increase the size of the herds, thus raising national tax revenue (both from customs charges on export sales and from the annual per capita tax on each pastoralist's herd). To reinforce this, the boreholes were located in such a way that the nomads would be nearer the towns, and hence under greater administrative and fiscal control.

Nobody is sure how many cattle there were in the Sahel, but livestock numbers probably did increase. Between 1938 and 1970, official statistics estimate that cattle herds in Niger rose three quarters of a million to four and a half million. During the same period, the figures show that the number of sheep and goats in that country increased from three million to nine million. Heavy overgrazing occurred around the new boreholes, and the Sahelian drought of 1968–1973 precipitated a crisis in which many herds died – but mainly from hunger,

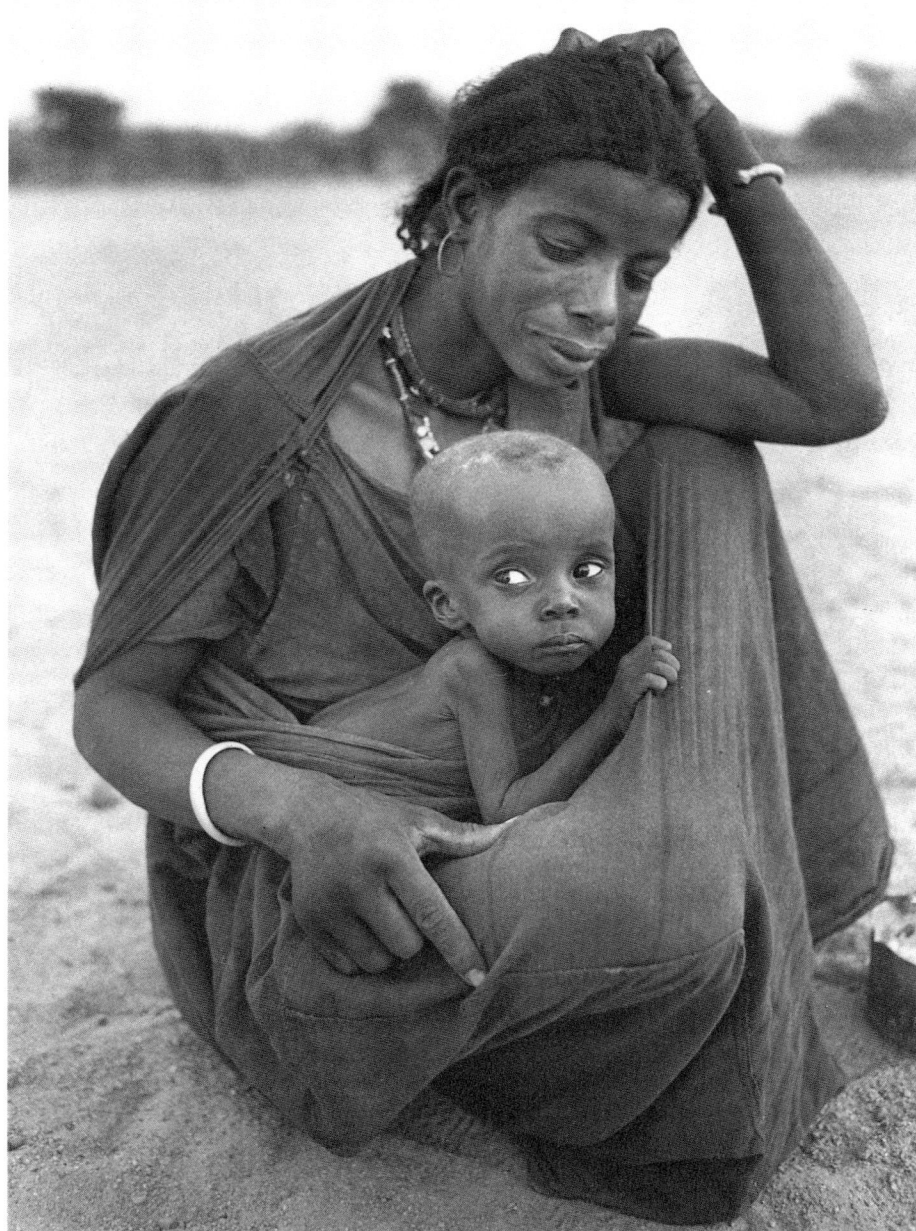

not water shortage.

Most attempts by Sahelian governments, backed by western funds, to get the nomads to adopt settled lifestyles have failed; no group will readily relinquish its culture and history. The problem the nomads have now and for the future is how to find more food for the cattle without further degrading the environment. The low, and decreasing, fertility of the soils in the remaining pastureland determines the limit of the herd sizes. The death of animals from shortage of grazing highlights the precarious nature of the nomads' position. Until the needs of their system are understood, and integrated into agricultural development plans, their survival chances cannot be assured.

Survival strategies of the poor

According to the World Bank, 90 per cent of the world's absolute poor still live in rural areas. In the Sahel, as the environment deteriorates under pressure, people have a growing need for cash with which to buy the food they cannot grow. One option has been to migrate in search of seasonal labour on the cocoa, coffee and pineapple plantations in the Ivory Coast and Ghana. Ghana's economic problems mean that its economy no longer has jobs to offer, but every year 500,000 people from Burkina Faso migrate to the Ivory Coast in search of work. Up to 100,000 of them never return.

The Ivory Coast bubble has now burst, and the country has one of the highest per capita debt commitments in Africa. Most of the debts were incurred during the boom years of the 1970s, when cocoa and coffee prices were relatively high. The government borrowed large amounts to finance expanding state structures, as well as expensive prestige projects. The country's growth rate owed much to migrant labour – by 1970, almost 45 per cent of the Ivory Coast population was of foreign origin. But commodity prices fell and imported oil costs

32

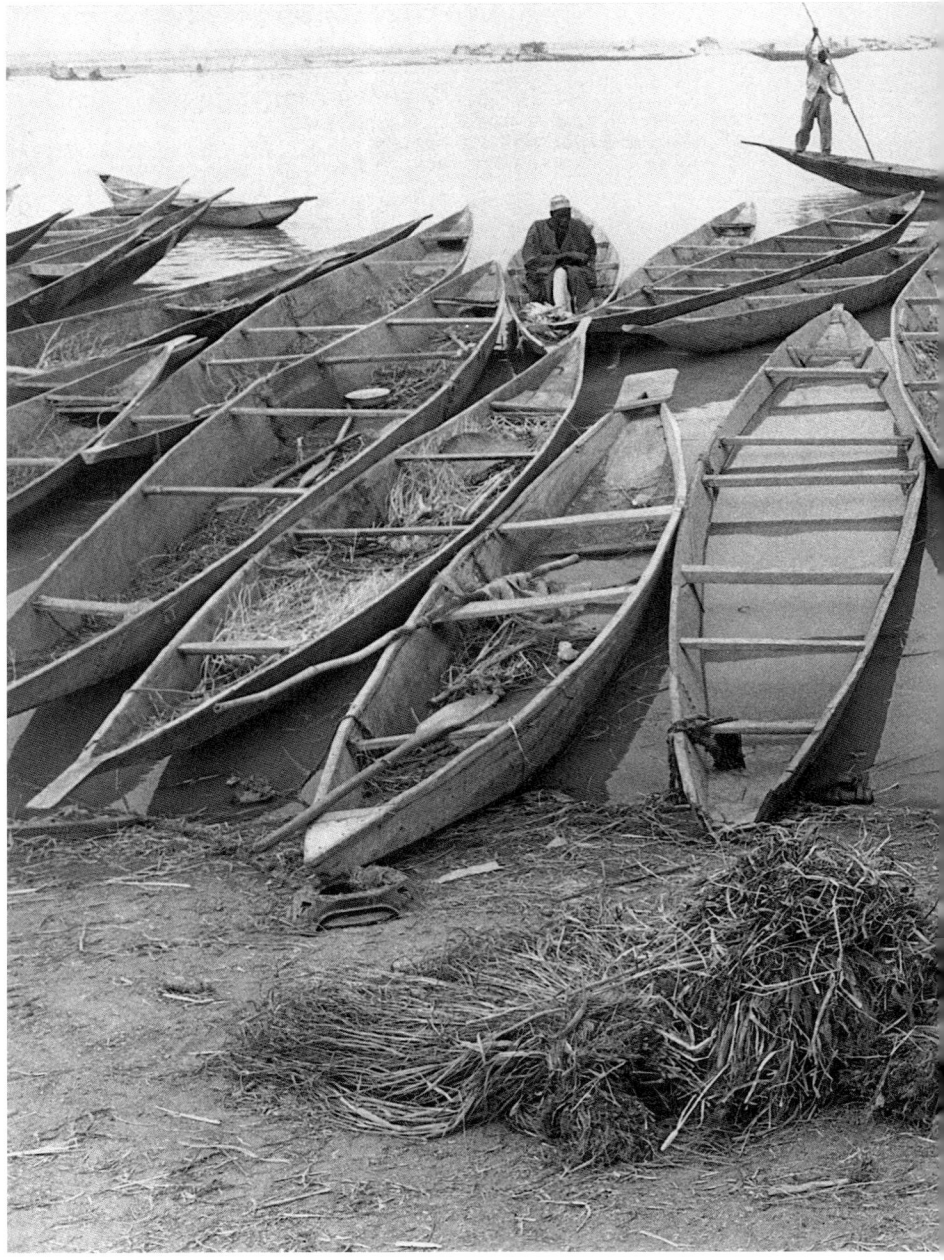

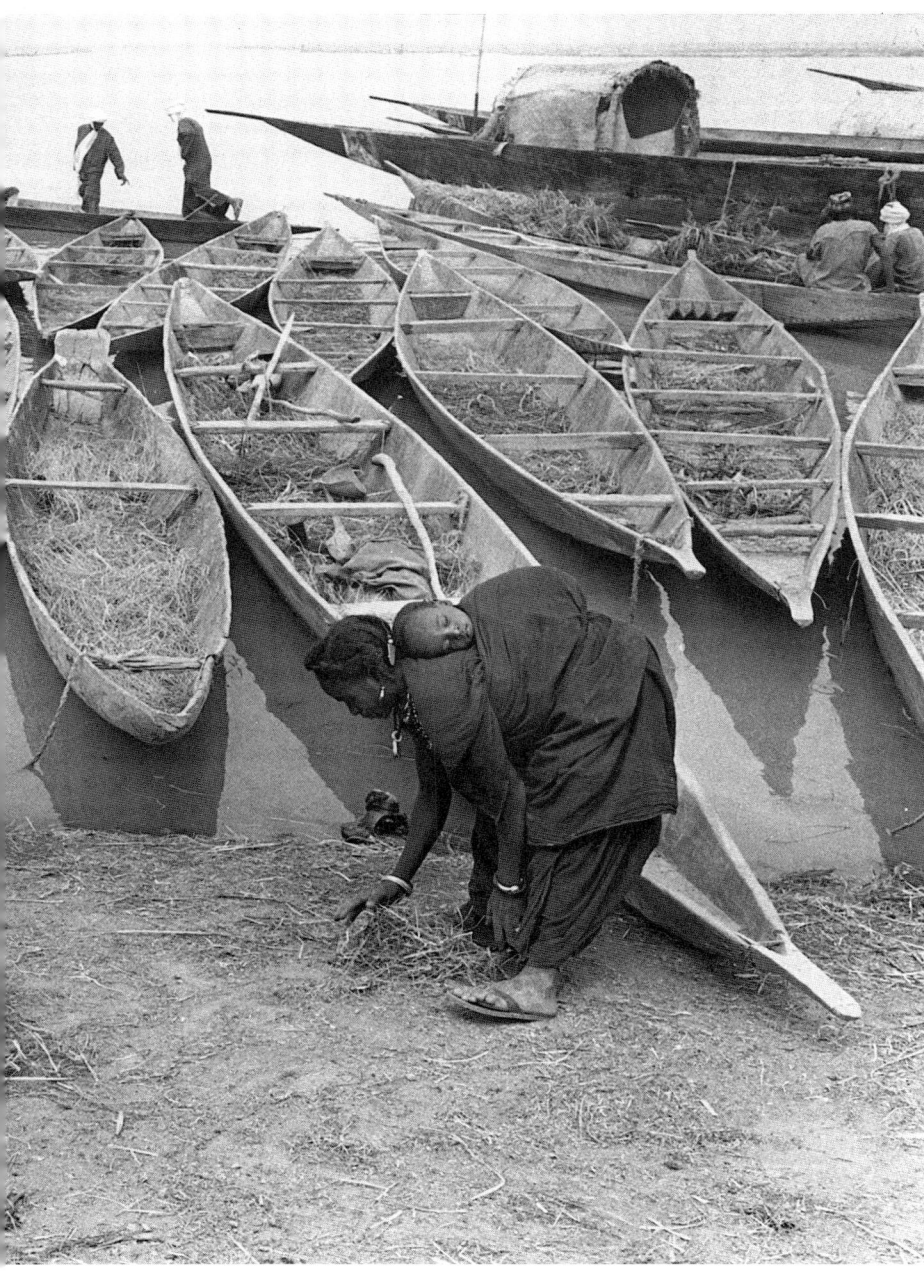

rose. The now-settled Sahelian labour force provides a natural scapegoat for the economic crisis, and could face expulsion, as did the immigrant workforces of West Germany and Nigeria.

Even with a wage from the plantations, most families do not have enough. They may respond by selling small animals such as sheep and goats, which function as 'walking banks' for the poor. Small-scale trading is important in the lives of the Sahel's rural poor, and those who lack the capital necessary to buy commodities in bulk resort to collecting wild fruit or wood from the bush to sell.

The months immediately before the harvest are the most difficult and hungry, and many people are forced to weed a wealthier farmer's fields for money. The implications of this are obvious; weeding on their own fields is reduced as a result, and the next harvest is likely to be smaller still as the crop is choked with weeds. A process is set in motion which culminates in the creation of a class of landless labourers. One farmer in Burkina Faso put it like this: 'Once the famine has caught up with you, you can never escape'.

The Sahel is still one of the least urbanized areas of the world, but more and more people are drifting to the towns. As in most of the poor countries, the capacity of the Sahel's small industrial sector to absorb this new-found workforce from the country-side is strictly limited. The function of the cities is likely to remain administrative and commercial, not industrial. The jobs do not exist. There are none on the horizon. More and more Sahelian peasants are leaving their homes for ever longer periods, not because wage labour is giving them access to a world of western-style consumption, but because poverty is driving them out of their villages.

A woman searches the ground for stray stalks of rice dropped by farmers bringing in their harvest to sell in the market at Gao.

33

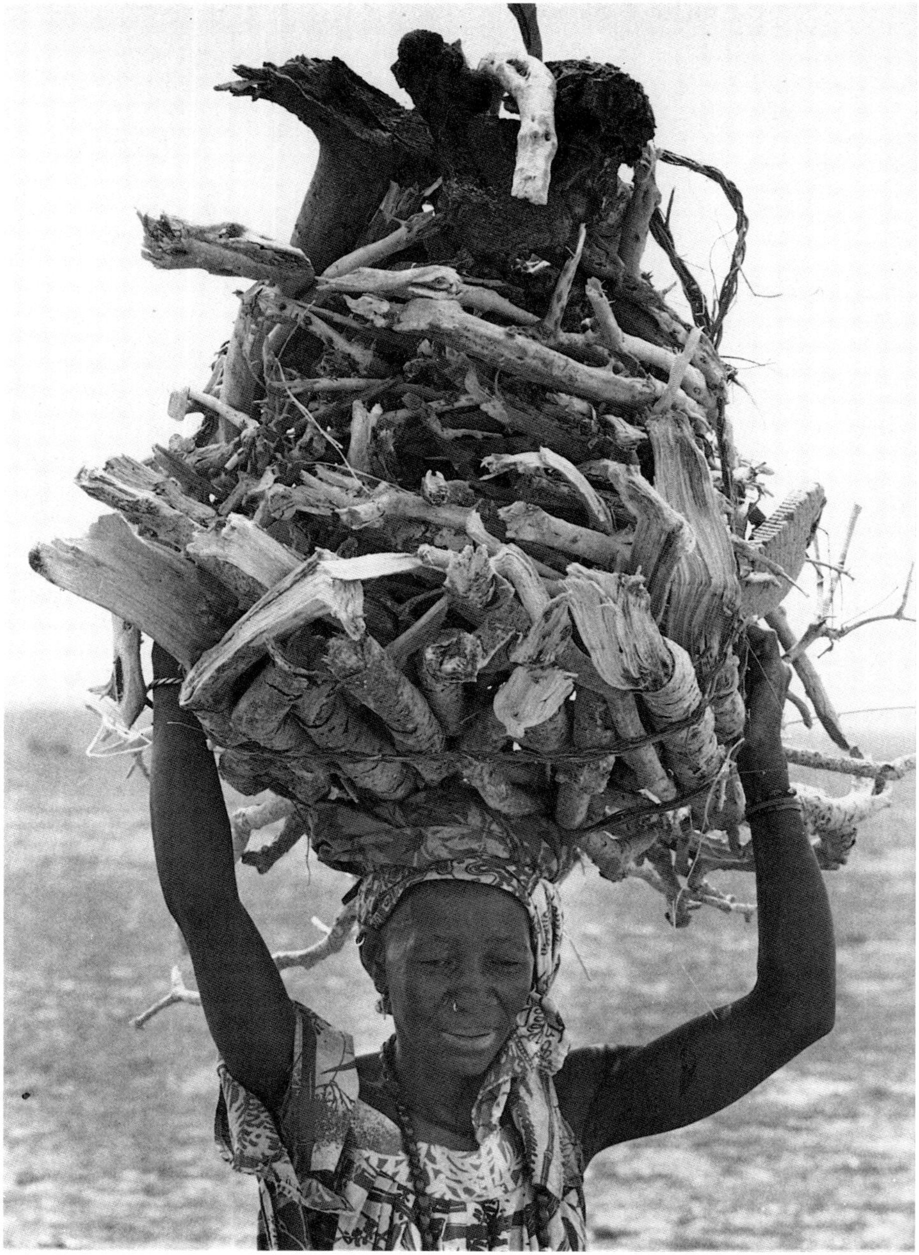

34

Selling firewood is a traditional way for the poorest to make some money. People used to gather only dead wood for sale but now deforestation forces them to fell live trees, so that the environment inevitably deteriorates.

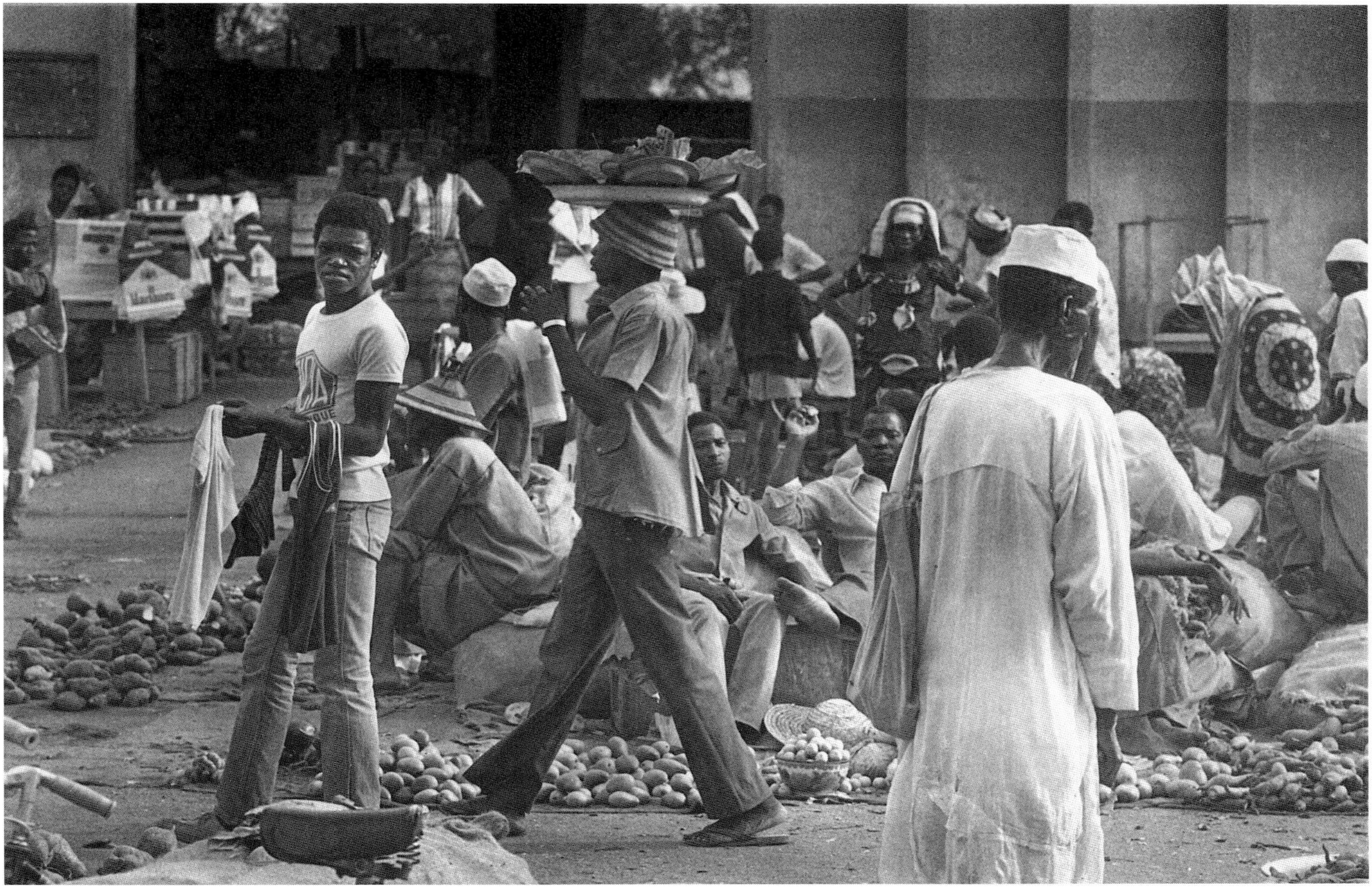

A market in Ouagadougou, Burkina Faso.
As conditions in the countryside get
worse, more and more people try to scrape
a living in the towns.

In the field of development, probably the most useful forms of assistance have come from the small non-governmental organizations. Many of these have recognized the causes of the process of impoverishment in the Sahel, and made serious attempts to devise projects which serve the interests of the poorest.

There is a danger that inter-governmental aid, in the final analysis, is more likely to serve the interests of the recipient government itself than that government's population. The interests of the two are unlikely to correspond. The mass of the population need, at the very least, mechanisms through which to prevent the deterioration of their economic and ecological life, so that they can continue in rural self-sufficiency. Governments need currency, preferably hard, with which to expand the state machinery, fuel urban economies and keep their hold on power. The source of this currency is, of course, the peasants and their land. The NGOs, relatively unfettered by the needs of governments to maintain the status quo, are evolving projects which have the interests of the local communities as their starting point.

For the most part, these programmes are not based on any romatic ideas of preserving the rural peasantry in isolation. They are directed towards giving the poor greater control over the way their lives are integrated into the national and international economy.

The schemes are based on the communities' own perceptions of their needs and problems, rather than those of foreign experts.

One illustration of contrasting approaches to a similar problem can be seen in two programmes aiming to halt soil erosion. In Burkina Faso, the state-controlled agency 'Rural Development Funds' is working on the problem. First, it sends a topographer to measure a preselected site, and determine the contour lines. Tractors then arrive in the village to construct small dykes which will prevent rainwater running off with the topsoil. Rich and poor peasants alike can benefit from such a scheme, but it is expensive and therefore limited by the agency's budget. More importantly, the end result is that farmers come to think that the solution to the problem of erosion lies with tractors and experts, and is beyond their grasp. Short-term results of the programme are impressive, but by taking the initiative out of the hands of the villagers, the long-term problem remains.

Small-scale projects based in the villages can have a better chance of long-term success than large technical development schemes. Ditches being dug here by villagers will irrigate their land with water taken from the river Niger by small diesel pumps, using technology that the people are able to control and maintain.

36

Reversing the process

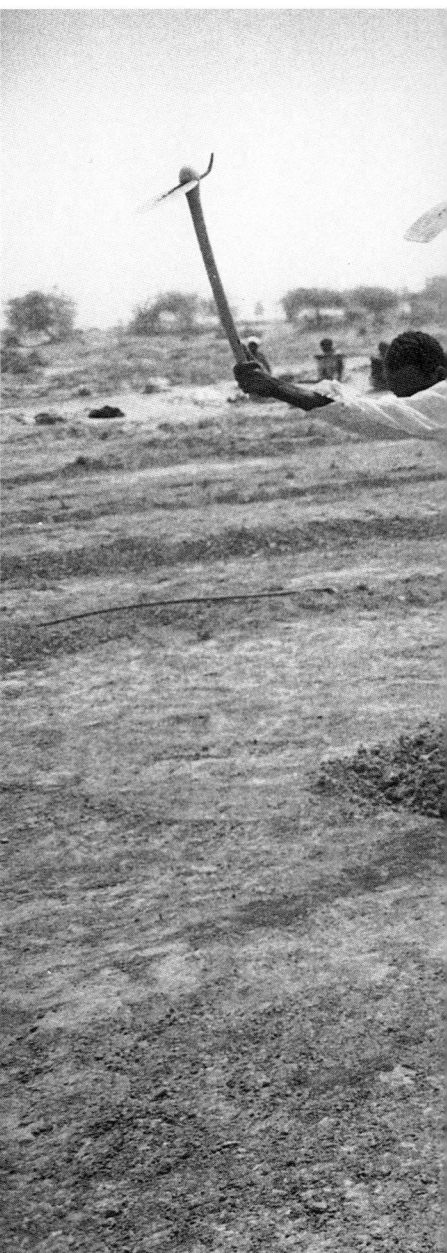

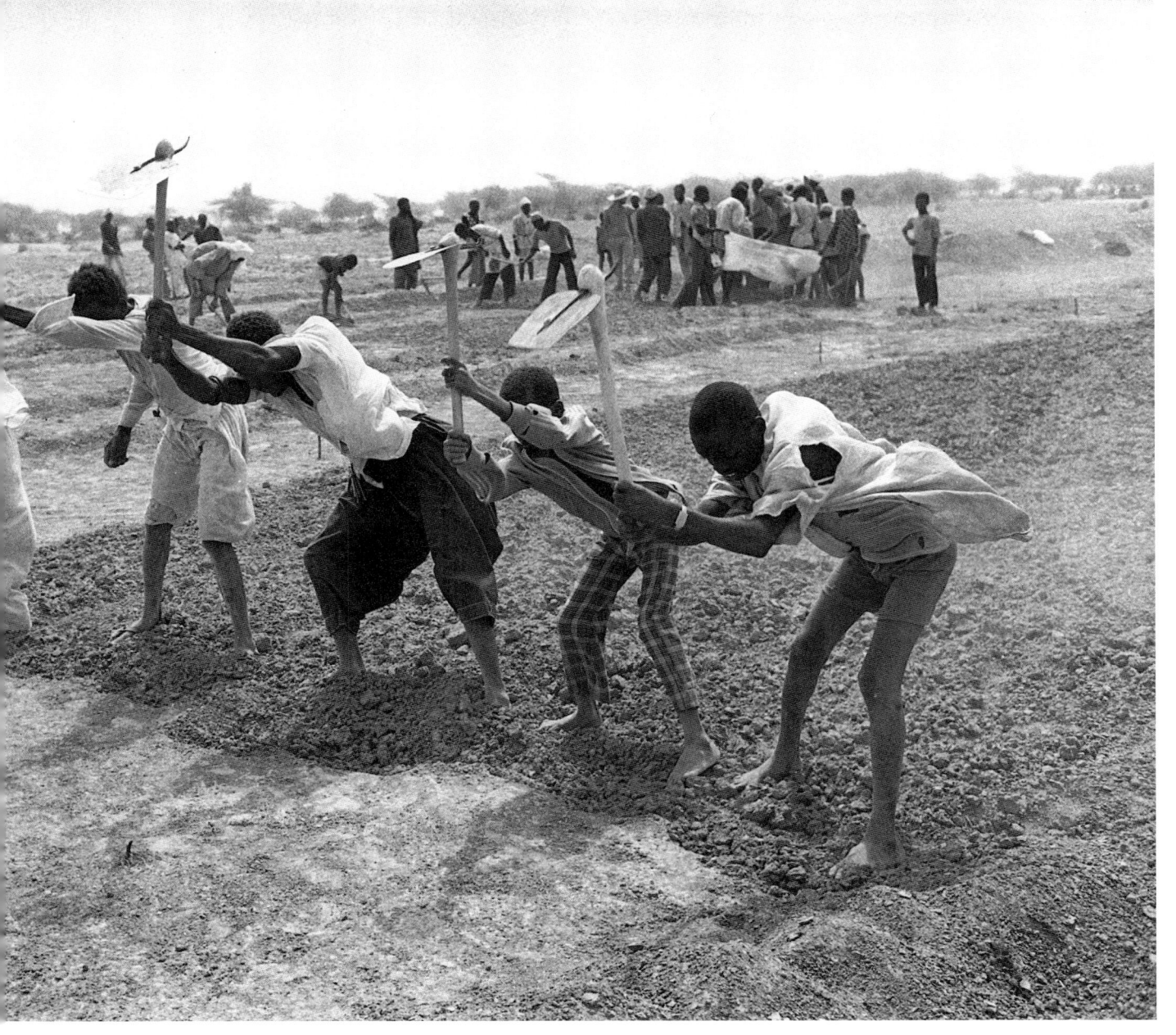

In contrast, another project in northern Burkina Faso aims to teach all farmers basic anti-erosion dyke construction techniques. These small dykes, built during the dry season from millet stalks, stones or other local materials, run along the contour lines of the farmers' fields and, just as in the other programme, prevent the rain rushing off the slope with the precious topsoil. But it is the peasants who work out the position of the contour line, using a transparent plastic tube filled with water as a spirit level, and build the dykes accordingly.

Although the basic idea behind this programme – that people should take responsibility for helping themselves – represented a significant step forward in development terms, project workers soon discovered that they were working primarily with the richer farmers. One reason was that during the dry season, when the work was carried out, many of the poor migrated to look for work on the Ivory Coast plantations. It was also explained by the fact that the dykes required a significant amount of labour. Having a sizeable and available labour force in itself implies a certain wealth. Some hired a team of young men from the village, trained by the project, to do the work on their fields in return for food. But as we have seen, poor families often do not have enough to feed themselves, let alone a group of labourers.

More often than not it is the fields of the poorest peasants which are most in need of anti-erosion schemes, since they tend to be the lowest quality and hardest worked land. The project therefore revised its approach. They introduced a food loan scheme whereby the project lends food to the poorer farmers who wish to hire labourers, and the farmers then use that food to feed the people who help them to construct their dykes. They must repay the food with interest to the project at harvest time. This is meeting with some success, although the very poorest people in the area are still afraid to borrow food when they habitually fail to produce enough for themselves.

Grain banks

Throughout the Sahel, the cereals market is dominated by private traders who are amongst the most efficient operators in Africa. They buy food at harvest time at the lowest possible price and then resell it at the highest possible price later in the year as shortages develop. Despite attempts by some Sahelian governments to regulate the market, private traders are not a social service, and it would be unrealistic to expect them to make lower profits voluntarily. Research into some markets has shown how the traders co-operate by agreeing the sale price of grain between themselves. State marketing boards sell grain in urban areas at controlled prices, mainly as a sop to the civil servants and army personnel on whom many regimes rely for their continued hold on power. The rural peasants who constitute the mass of the poor are unable to meet the traders' prices, and have no grain available to them at a wholesale price.

In an attempt to combat this, the idea of village level cereal banks was revived in Burkina Faso just after the last drought, and has now begun to spread widely in the Sahel. This system was commonplace in pre-colonial Africa but broke down under heavy taxation by the Europeans. A village co-operative group raises funds, usually a loan, from a non-governmental organization, with which to buy grain at harvest time when the price is low. They may either purchase it from within their own village, or from elsewhere in the country if their own harvest was poor. The co-op constructs a small grain store, and keeps the food for six to eight months until members of the group have begun to run out of food from their own field, and market prices have risen. The group then decides at what price the grain should be sold, bearing in mind inflation and the need to repay the initial loan.

Technically, the idea is very sound, and considerable amounts of money have been invested by donors in this form of food security. But the idea has spread so fast that often the actual workings of such co-ops have not been examined in enough detail by their sponsors. A doctoral student recently spent several months studying just one bank in the village of Cooksin in Burkina Faso, and came up with some disturbing conclusions. The poor households in the village were not members of the co-op. In the main, grain was bought from the bank by comparatively rich households, perhaps to resell at a profit. Four of the six members of the cereal bank committee came from these richer households, and they determined who was able to buy the controlled price grain. Furthermore, the grain was only sold in 100 kilo sacks, a quantity which the poor can rarely afford to buy. When they did buy it, it was by taking credit from the bank, which they had to repay in kind after the following harvest at a rate of interest of 20 per cent. In short, in that particular village, the economic benefits to the poor were minimal, while the advantage gained by the better-off households allowed them to consolidate their position by buying more agricultural materials and hiring labour.

This kind of problem is relatively easy to overcome once it has been identified. But it illustrates why the non-governmental organizations need to spend as much time learning how the village hierarchy works as they spend on determining the nature of their projects. The latter cannot be successfully set in motion before a social understanding has been reached. And it seems necessary to take as a starting point the fact that if the intervention is economically advantageous, then the dominant group within the community will attempt to hijack it, and in all probability will be well placed to do so.

38

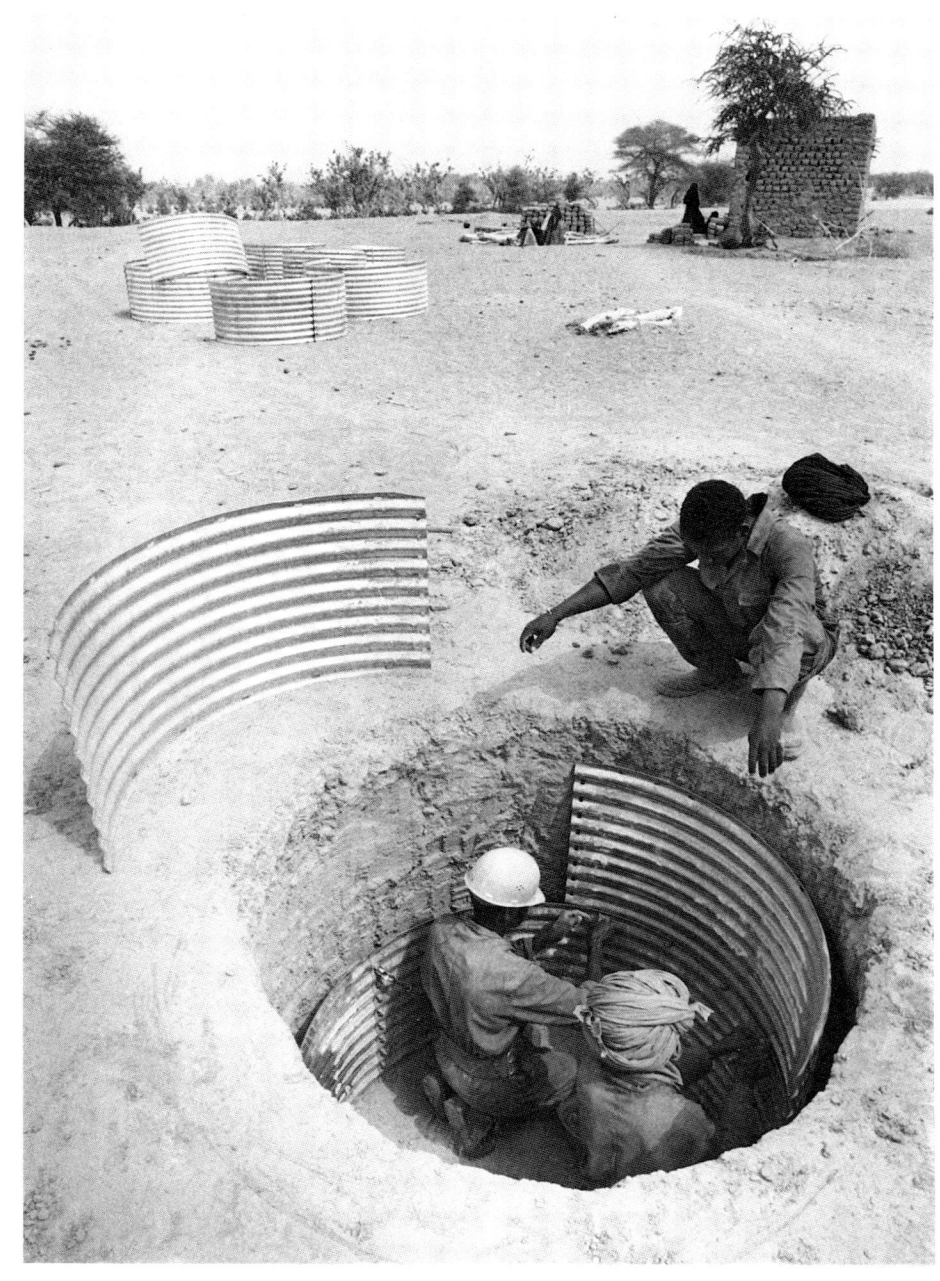

Control of water supplies means life or death at the edge of the desert. Successful NGO water projects let the communities concerned decide where the well should be located. In this case, in the remote area of Kidal in Northern Mali, the people chose a site where pastureland has been under-used because of the lack of watering points for animals.

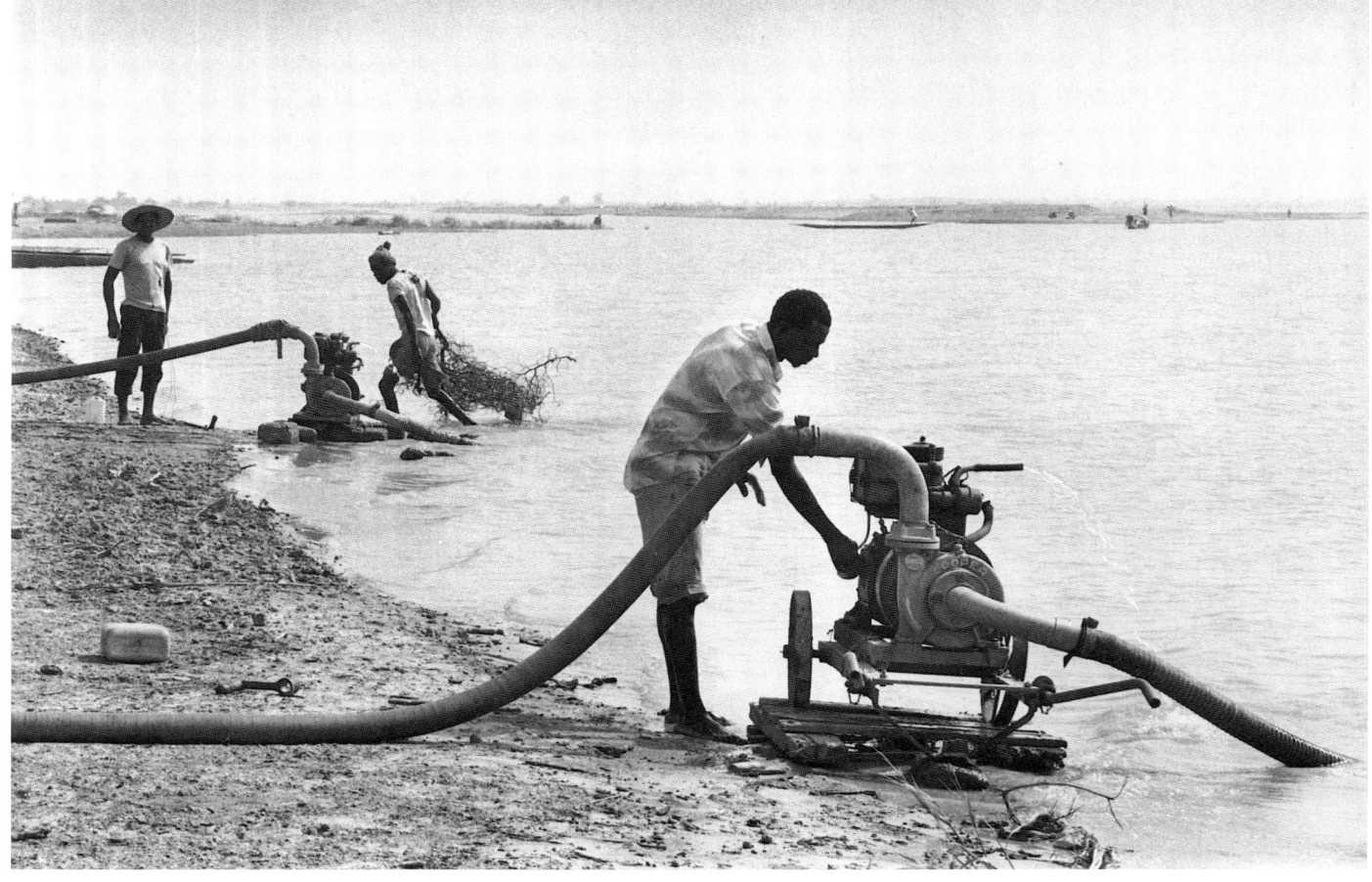

**Small-scale irrigation pumps on the river
Niger at Diré.**

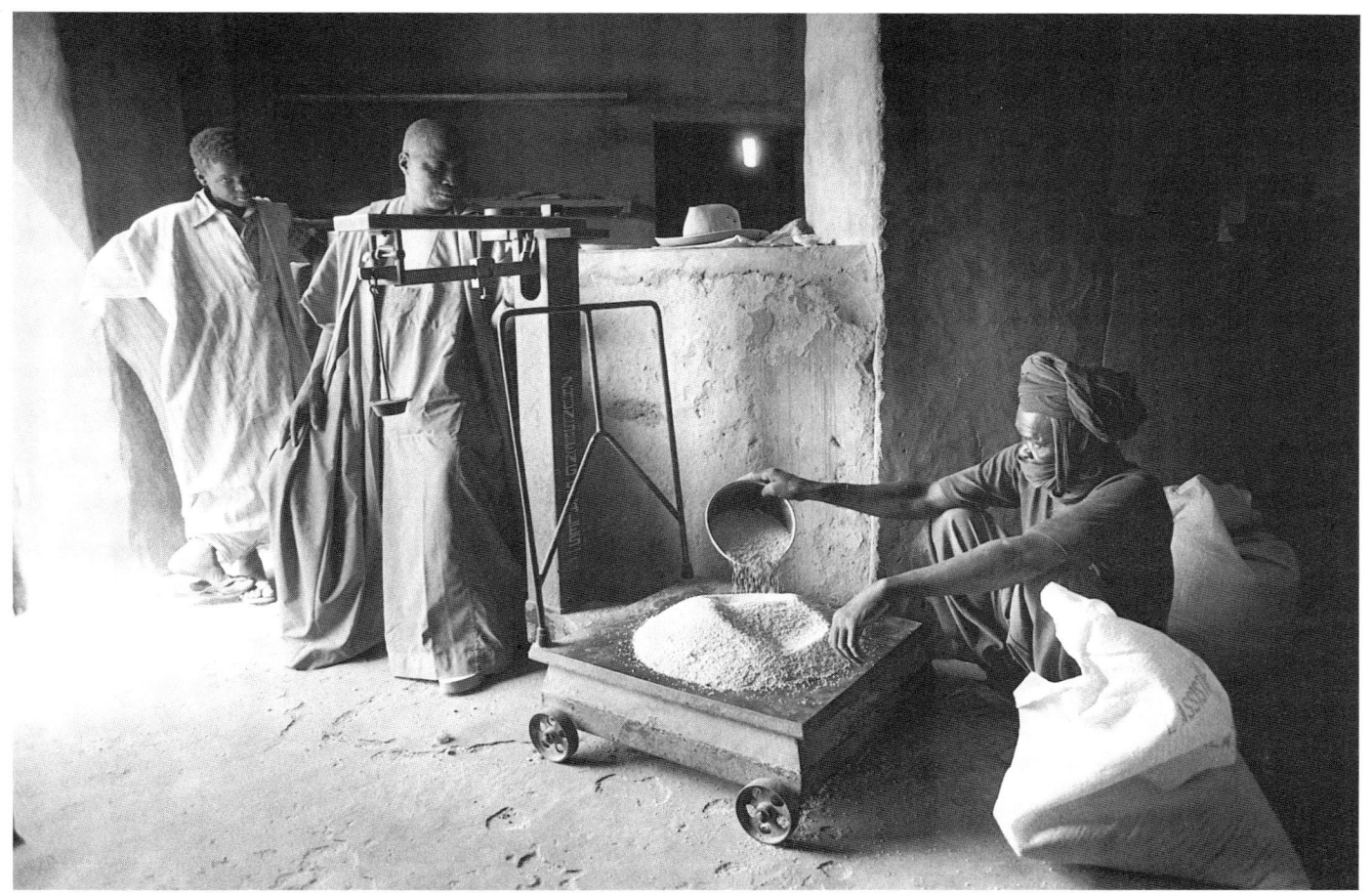

Farmers' co-operatives, like this one in
Kidal, northern Mali, help to maintain the
price of grain at an affordable level for
co-op members all the year round, and so
bypass profiteering traders.

Western governments donating food to be used in food-for-work programmes often give what is convenient and surplus, but not what is appropriate.

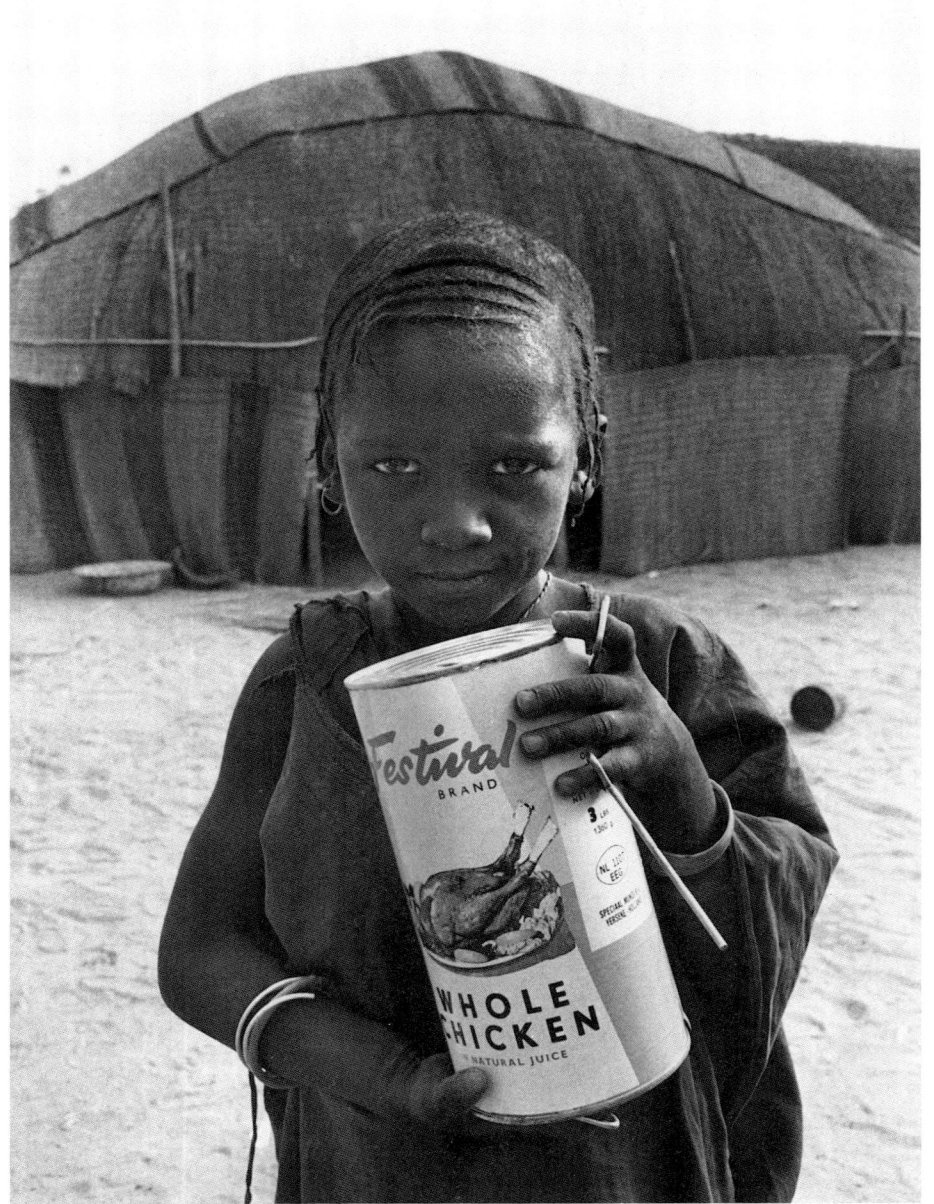

42

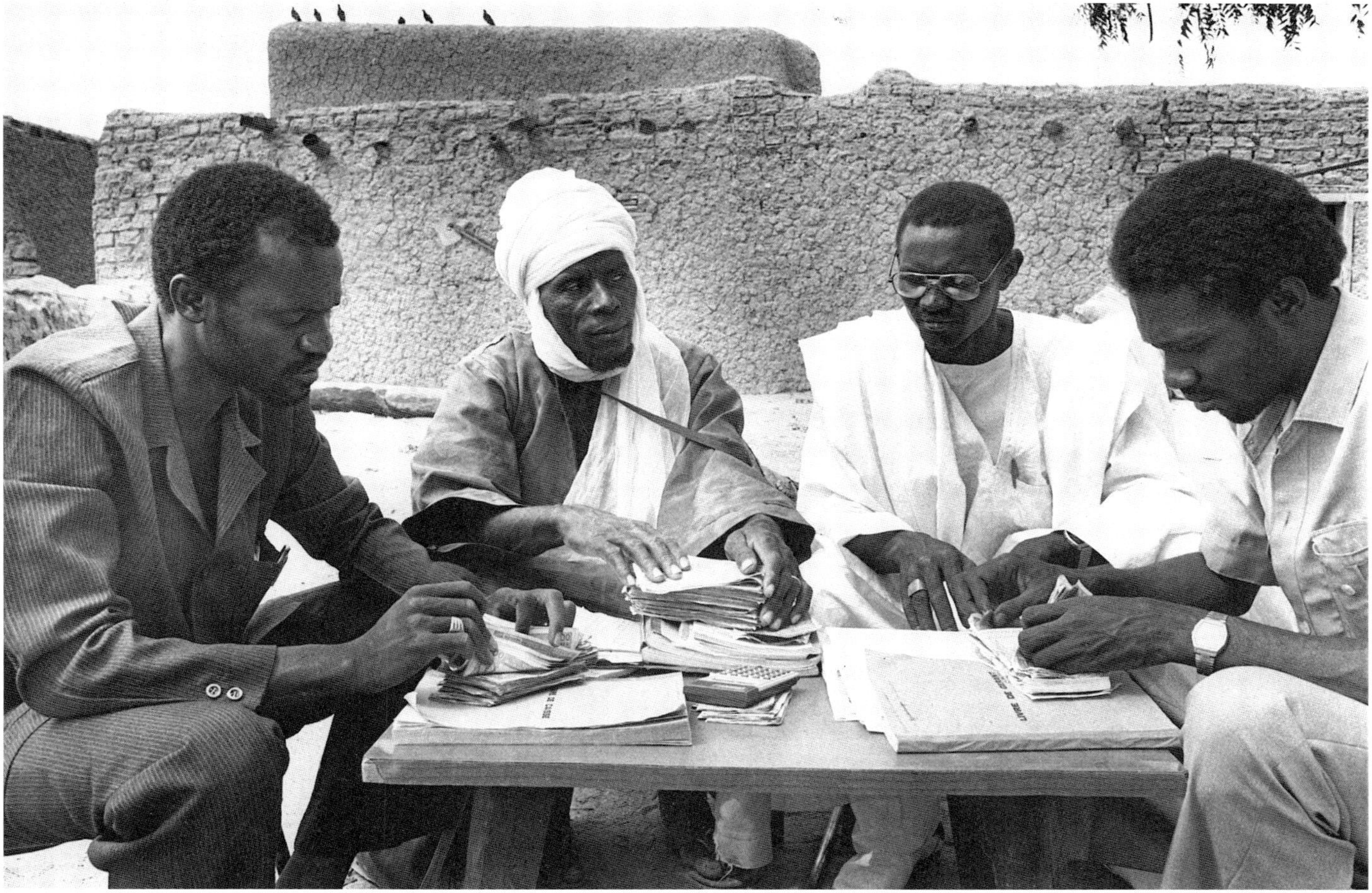

Co-op members record the accounts of
their grain transactions.

43

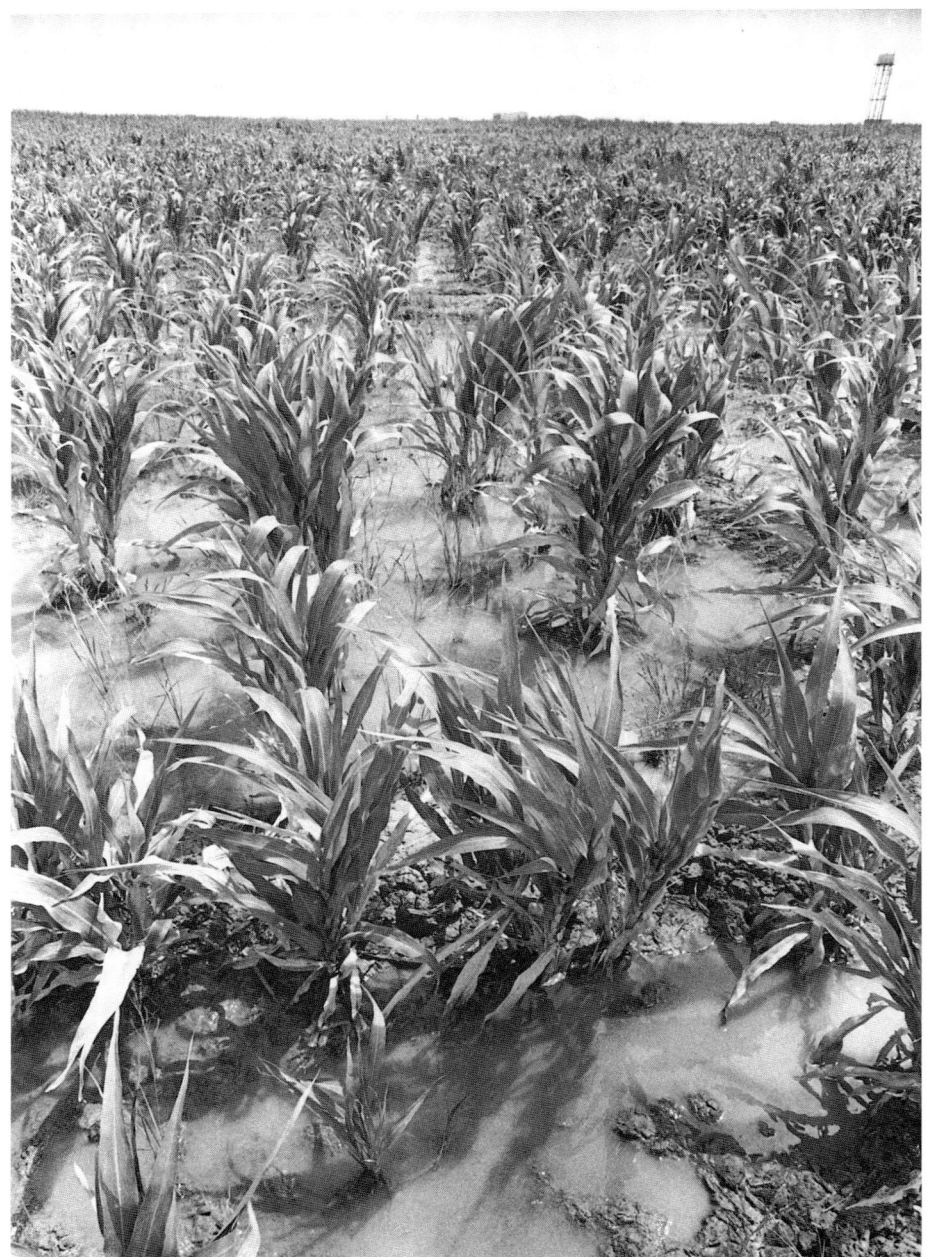

44

'An analysis of famine that puts the blame on an "encroaching desert" will never come to grips with the inequalities in power at the root of the problem. Solutions proposed will inevitably be limited to the technical and administrative aspects – irrigation programmes, modern mechanization, new seed varieties, foreign investment, grain reserve banks, and so on. Such an analysis allows no reflection upon the political and economic arrangements that, far more than changes in rainfall or even climate, are at the root of low productivity and human deprivation.'
Frances Moore Lappe
and Joseph Collins,
Food First

Young irrigated millet at Diré.

'The person who receives education is like a man who has been given all the food available in a starving village in order that he might have the strength to bring back supplies from a distant place.'
Julius Nyerere, President of Tanzania

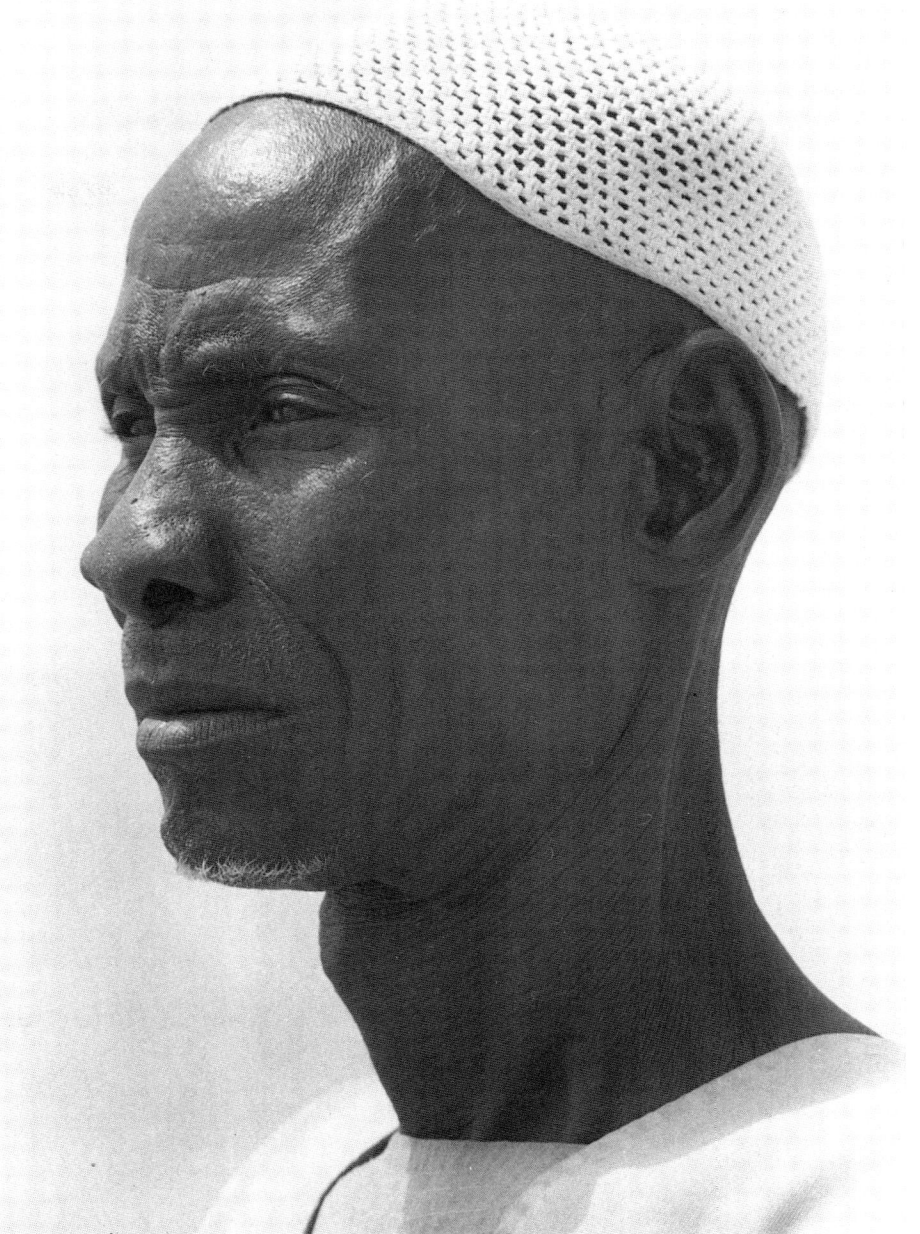

Malian river nomad.

46

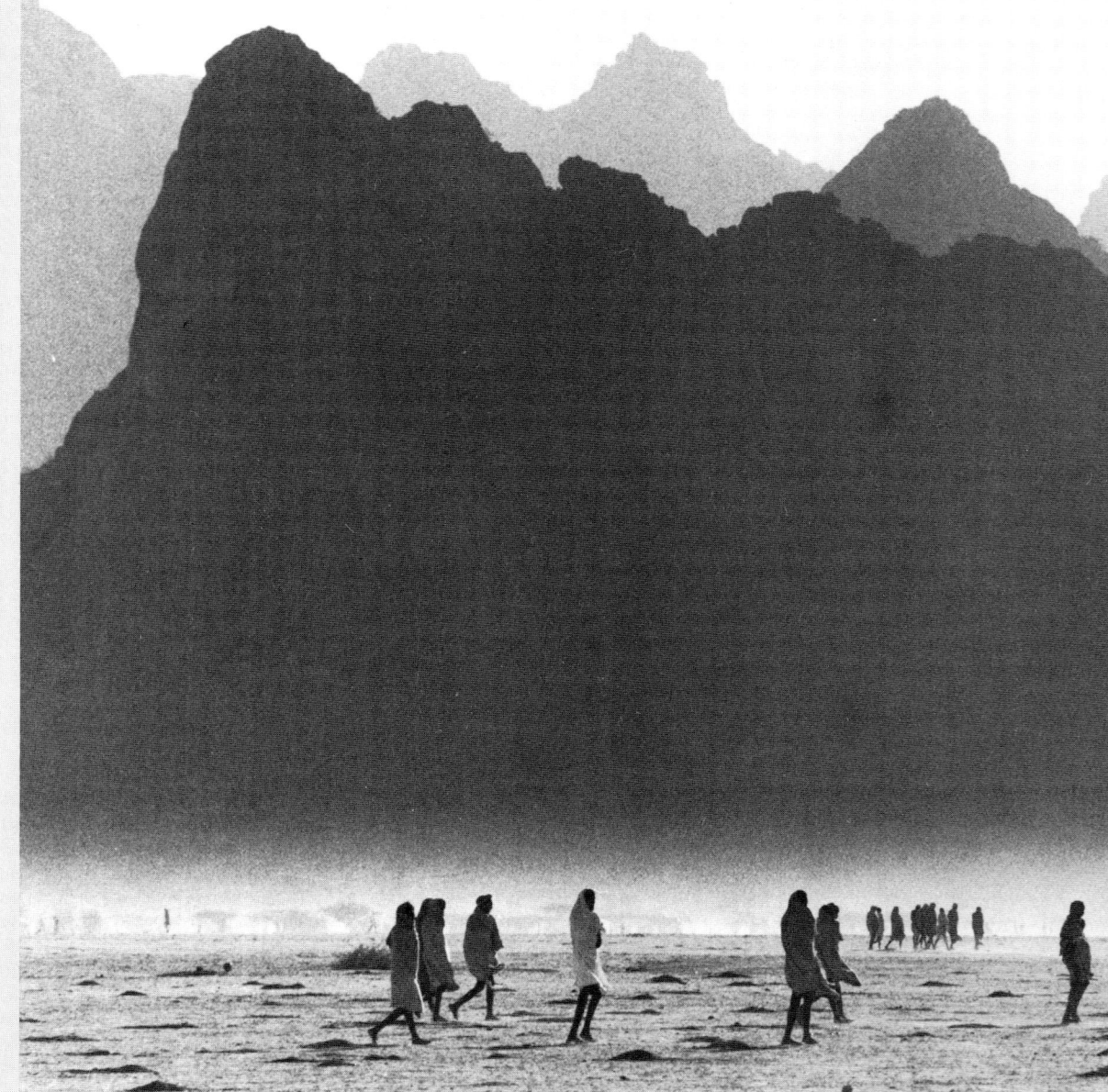

THE HORN
OF AFRICA

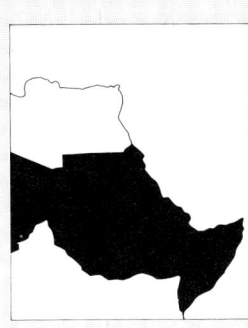

47

Sudan under President Jafar Numeiri was a prime target for Western aid. A former British colony, it stands between Libya and Ethiopia, and has had extremely bad relations with both countries. This was, of course, reassuring to the West. Under Numeiri, Sudan received about one quarter of all United States governmental aid to 'black Africa'. Numeiri's unpopular regime gained routine consignments from the US of PL480 food aid, which helped prevent social unrest, particularly in the capital, Khartoum.

In late 1984, hunger and disaffection prompted food riots all over Northern Sudan, many of them initiated by school-children whose state boarding schools were unable to feed them. At the end of March 1985, pressure from the IMF forced the Sudanese government to increase the price of bread and sugar, both staple foods. These price rises precipitated more riots in Khartoum, and Numeiri was deposed in an army-headed coup in April 1985. Sudan's new transitional government is moving towards a non-aligned position, and establishing better relations with Libya and Ethiopia, to the discomfort of its long-standing allies in Cairo and Washington.

The belief, prevalent in the 1970s, that Sudan could become the breadbasket of the Middle East seems bitterly ironic today. The country has been overtaken in recent years by many social and economic problems, including inflation, disinvestment, and the resurgence of the civil war being waged by the southern rebel movement against the northern establishment. 'Sudan tabaan – Sudan is tired', people say.

After Numeiri's introduction of Islamic Sharia law in September 1983, more than 200 people had their right hands amputated for theft, despite the fact that some of these 'thieves' were stealing in order to eat, a crime specifically exempted from punishment by the Koran. Many Sudanese were prompted to remark that under Numeiri's Sharia only small thefts were punished – large-scale corruption went unpunished.

Years of decline in the Sudan are partly attributable to the 'breadbasket strategy'. To rid itself of a dependence on the world market, based on the export of cotton and groundnuts, Sudan planned to grow food for export to the Arab region. Heavily supported by a few key Saudi Arabian entrepreneurs, the strategy rested on large-scale Arab investments in irrigation and the mechanization of cereals production.

But work did not progress as fast as had been planned, the cost of the imported equipment spiralled upwards in the late 1970s, and the Arab loans fell due before the projects were even completed. Sudan was left with no option but to take out short-term commercial balance of payments loans at high rates of interest. But banks would only lend the money if Sudan called in the IMF. The IMF recommended a rapid increase in cotton production to relieve the debt burden, which was by now extremely serious, and put together an 'economic rescue package'.

However, the cotton schemes' irrigation systems and agricultural machinery had not been maintained during the euphoric days of the 'breadbasket strategy'. Yields were low, and export earnings were badly hit by the continuing recession in world cotton prices. Sudan was unable to keep up with the interest payments on its debts, and the rescue package fell apart.

The year 1984 was the most disastrous ever for the Sudanese economy. Rising interest charges meant that, for the first time, Sudan was paying more for servicing its debts than it was earning from its exports. In the same year, oil exploration operations in the south of the country were halted as a result of rising instability in the south, and the oil to which Sudan and its creditors had been looking remained in the ground. The US bailed out the Sudan time and time again, but by late 1984 its patience was wearing thin.

For a decade in Sudan, large-scale development programmes have bypassed most of the population and have concentrated on expensive, import-dependent irrigation schemes. The Jonglei Canal, intended to boost the Nile waters by channelling the vast Sudd swamp, had been a planners' dream for a hundred years. When work finally started on the project in the late 1970s,

48

Sudan

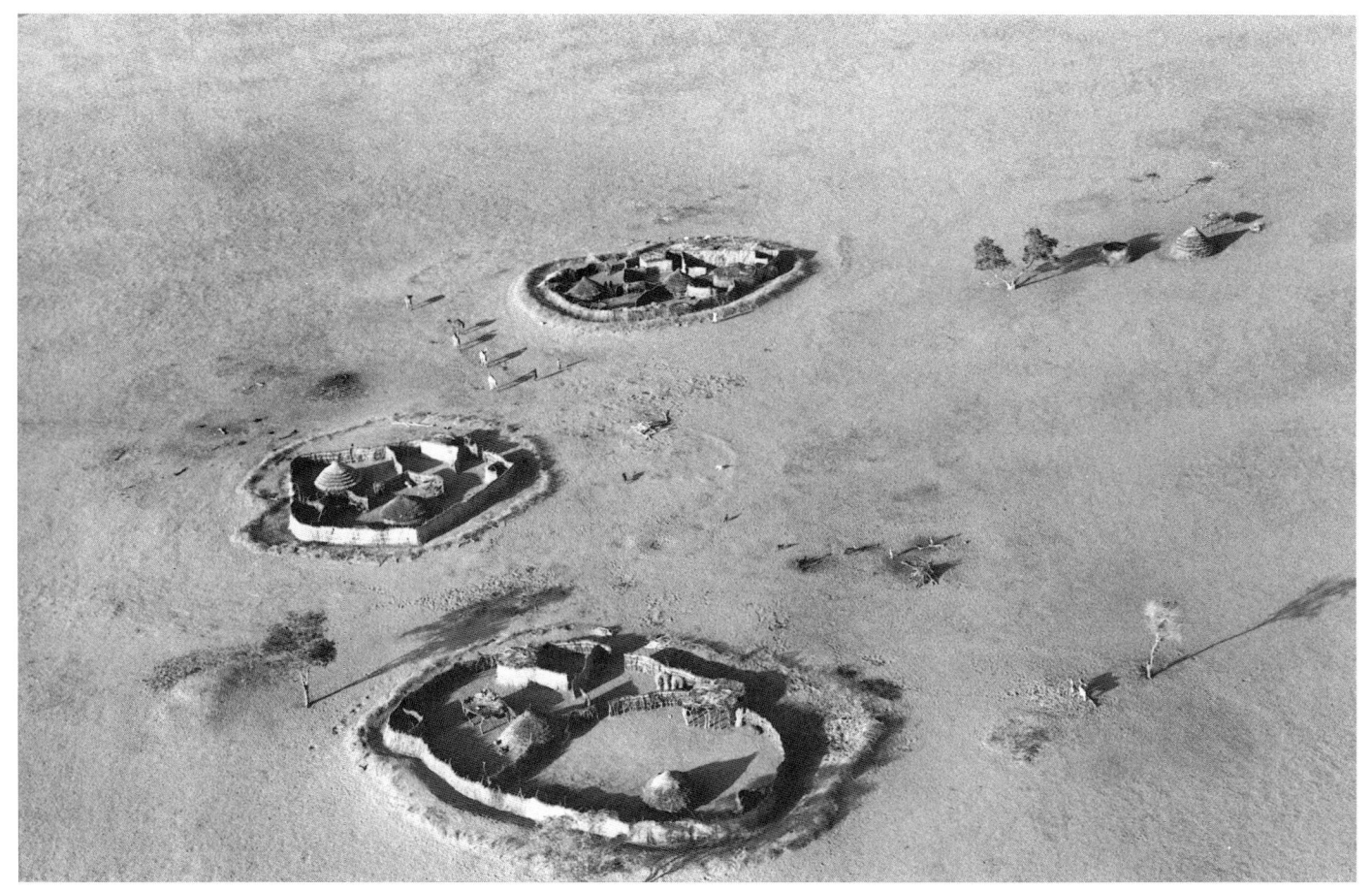

In Sudan, Africa's largest country, the predominantly rural population of peasant farmers and nomads is scattered over one million square miles. The terrain ranges from desert in the north to equatorial rainforest in the south. Here in Kordofan, western Sudan, the people have been hard hit by drought.

southern leaders claimed that it would benefit irrigation in Egypt and northern Sudan at the expense of local people. One of the first actions of the rebel southern movement, the Sudanese Peoples' Liberation Army (SPLA) was to kidnap nine employees of the French company building the canal in 1983. Included in their ransom demands was the order that work on the canal should cease. The largest single machine in the world, brought in to dig the canal, has stood idle since then.

Meanwhile, famine has taken hold of the Sudan. The arrival of up to 100,000 hungry nomads on the edge of the capital from regions in the west precipitated an awareness of the plight of the countryside amongst both the urban Sudanese and the world's press. The Sudanese government was slow to appeal for international assistance for its famine victims, and some observers explained this in terms of Numeiri's reluctance to accept the defeat of the breadbasket strategy.

Alarm bells were finally sounded on behalf of the Sudanese people in early 1985. An international relief effort was mounted, but the rainy season soon turned the operation into a logistical nightmare. Nyala, capital of the worst-affected region, lies 1,300 kilometres south west of Khartoum by rail. There is no all-weather road to the semi-desert Darfur region, inhabited by more than three million nomads and peasant farmers.

The single-track railway, under-financed for many years, proved unequal to the planned movement of 1,800 tonnes per day of emergency food rations to the west. By mid-1985, the US government and the EEC were considering parachuting grain into the most devastated areas. The number of dead could only be guessed at. People died in remote areas, invisible to both foreign relief workers and the Sudanese authorities. UNICEF estimated that only 10 per cent of those in immediate need of food were being reached. No such relief operation was attempted in the south of the country, parts of which have also been hit by drought.

The United Nations' newly-established emergency office for Africa requested $78 million in emergency funds for Sudan in 1985. But in the same year, Sudan was faced with a bill for $213 million for the interest charges on its foreign debts.

Sudan remains one of the poorest countries in the world, despite its agricultural potential. But now it has one of the highest debts per head of population in the world. The World Bank solution for Sudan is further liberalization of the economy, with more incentives to farmers, just as it is in Mali, on the other side of the continent. But, as President Nyerere of Tanzania has observed, such changes are not helpful to a peasant trying to feed the family from a barren patch of soil without fertilizer, tools or irrigation.

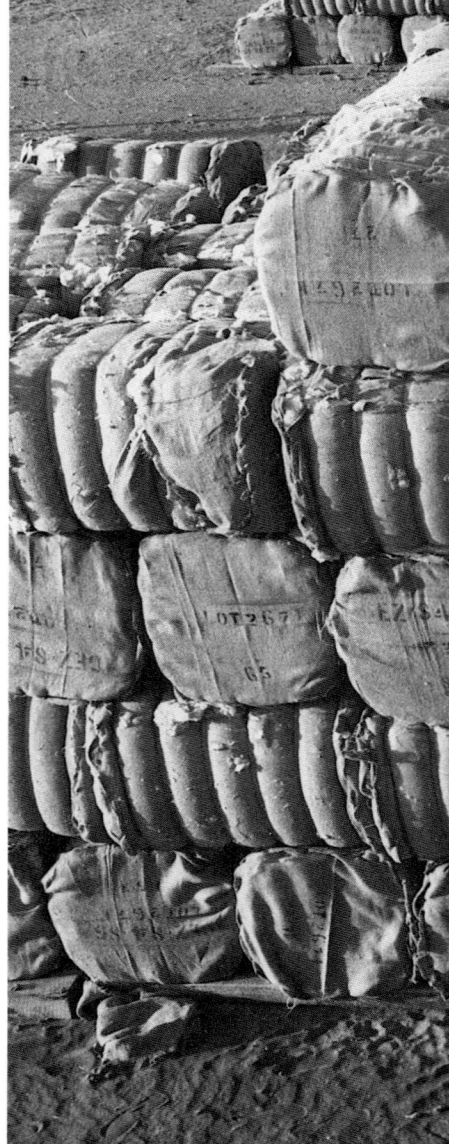

The Gezira scheme, run by the Sudanese government, uses water from the Nile to irrigate more than two million acres, making it the largest farm under one management in the world. Cotton, its main crop, earns 60 per cent of Sudan's foreign exchange, but this cannot keep up with the price of oil. Chronic petrol shortages afflict the whole country.

50

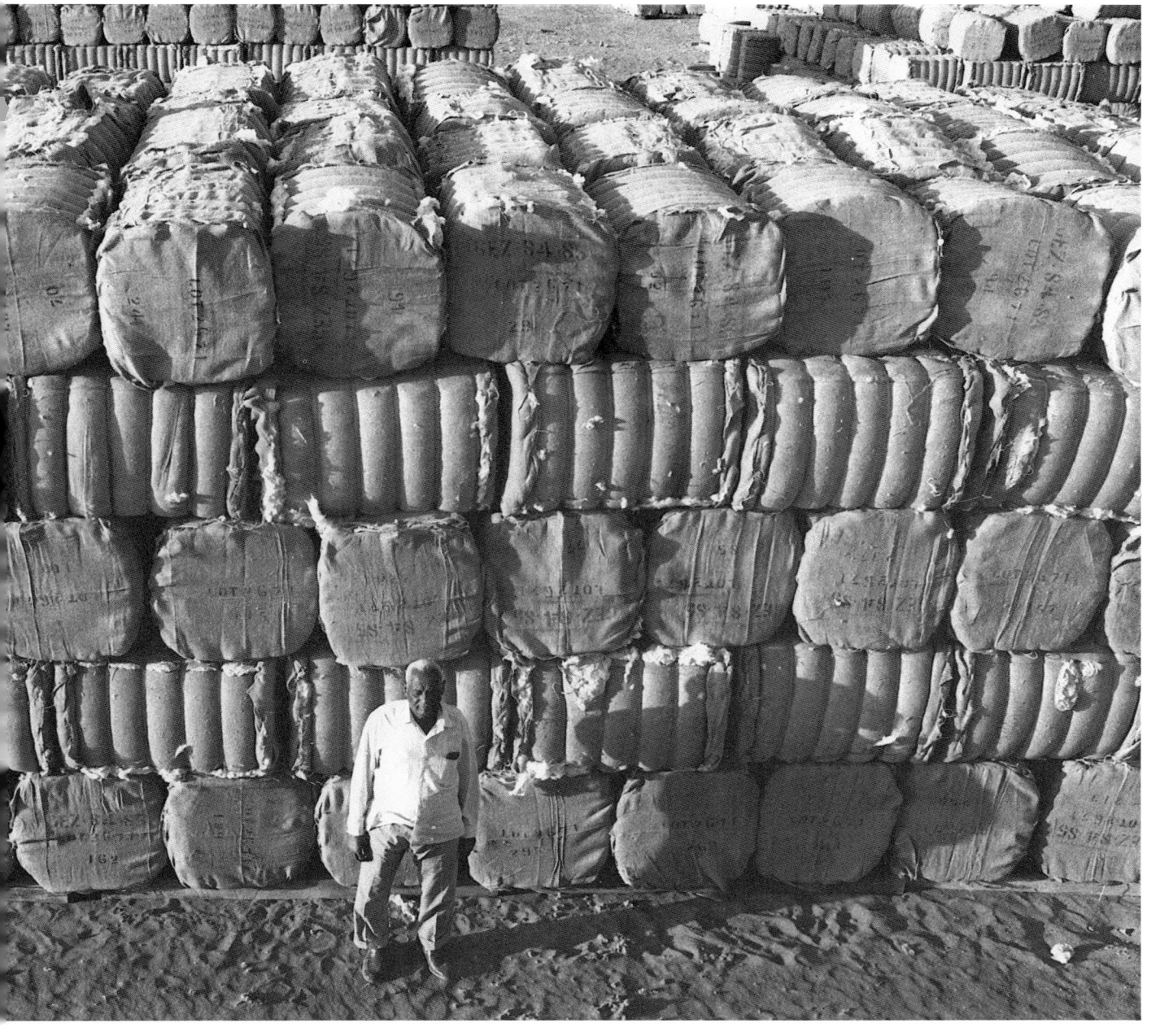

51

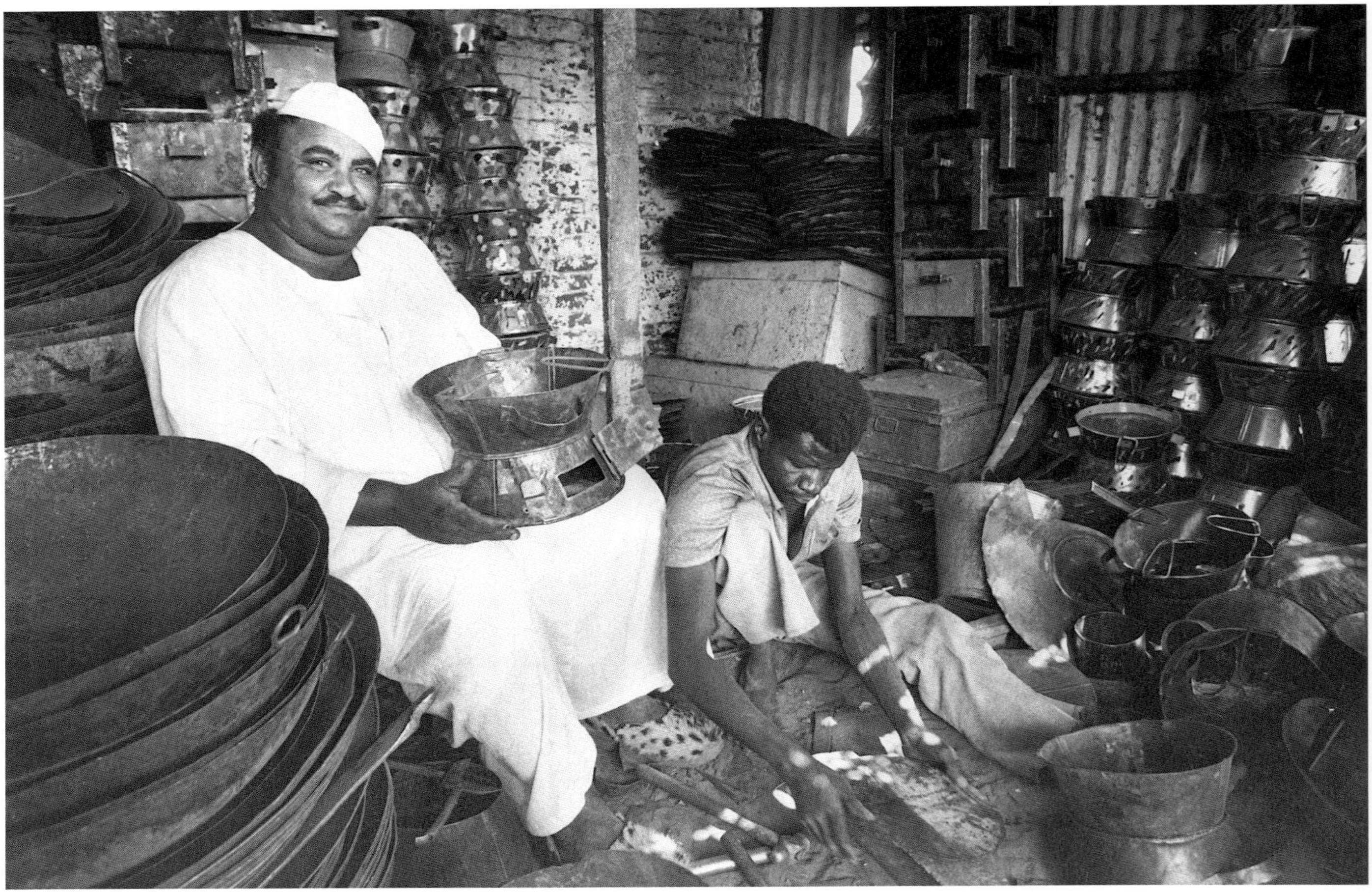

In the urban areas of Sudan, as elsewhere
in Africa, most people use charcoal for
cooking. Cutting wood to make charcoal is
a primary cause of deforestation. A 'fuel-
efficient' stove which uses 50 per cent less
charcoal than the conventional type has
been developed by an American NGO, and
is now being made commercially in local
markets. However, it can only have a
significant impact on halting deforestation
if its use becomes widespread.

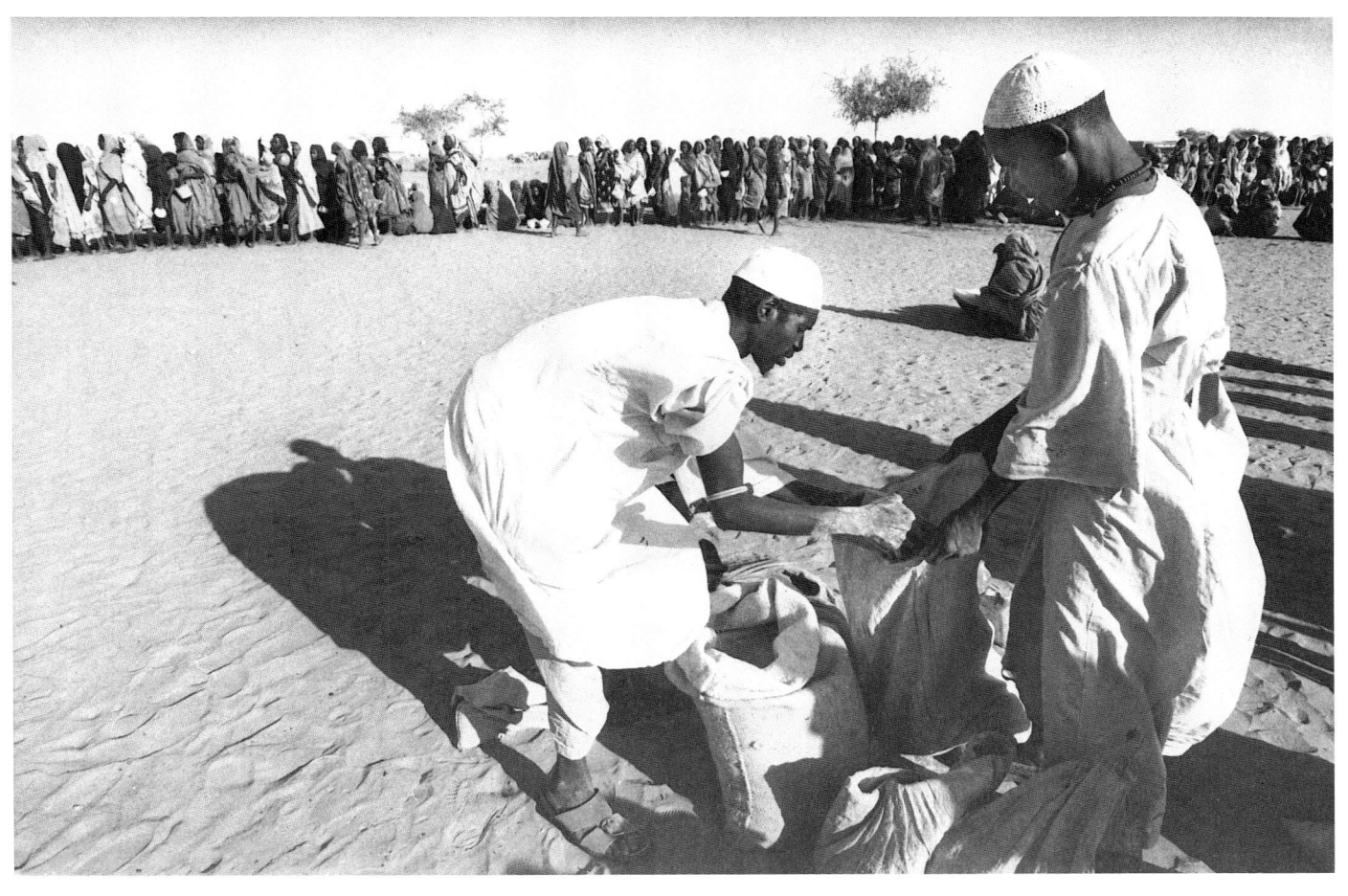

By late 1984, drought had forced many
thousands of Sudanese to leave their homes
in search of food. Here at a temporary
government relief camp at El Obeid, 27,000
people had gathered, hoping to receive
emergency rations of grain and milk.

54

Tigrayans fleeing the famine pick up their meagre possessions after a rest stop, and continue their journey over the mountains into Sudan.

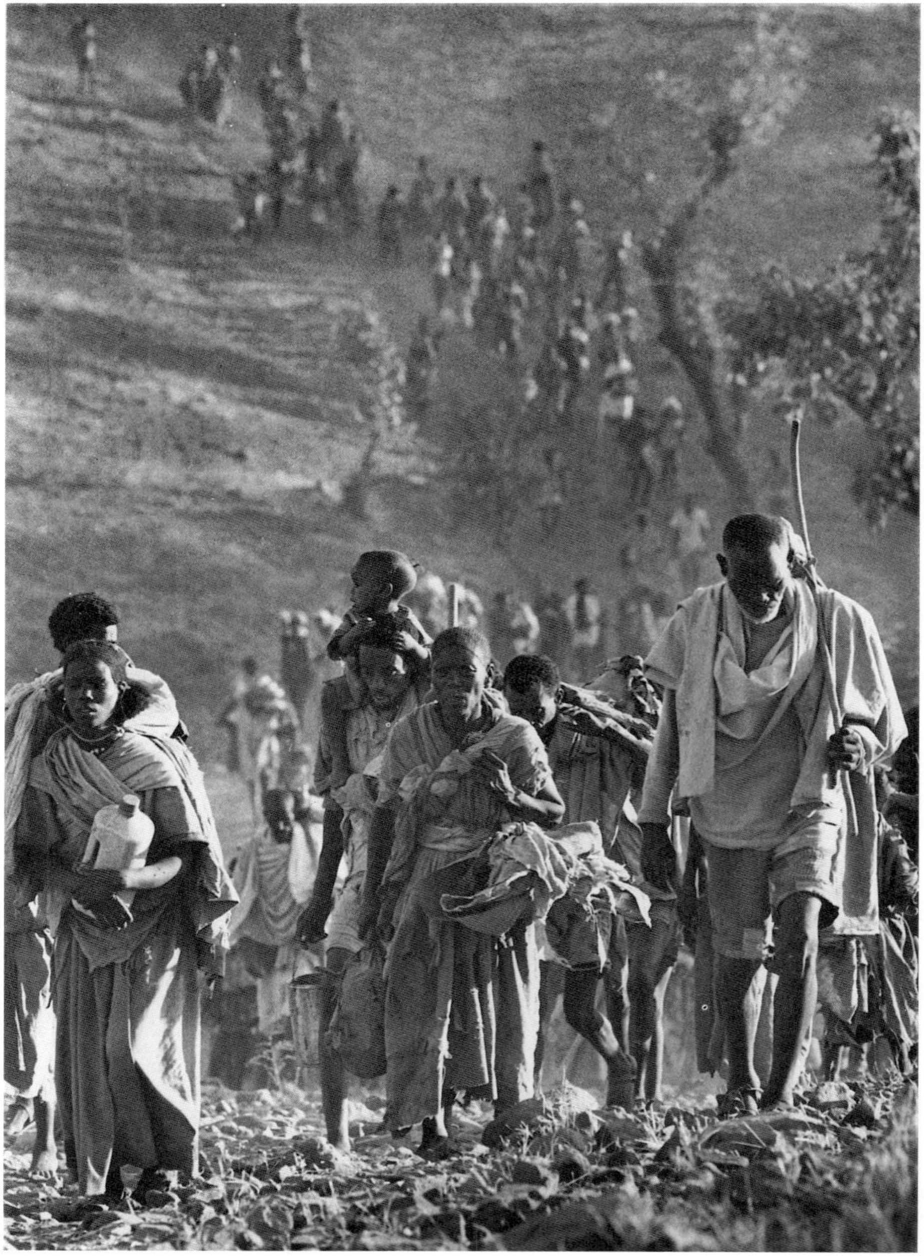

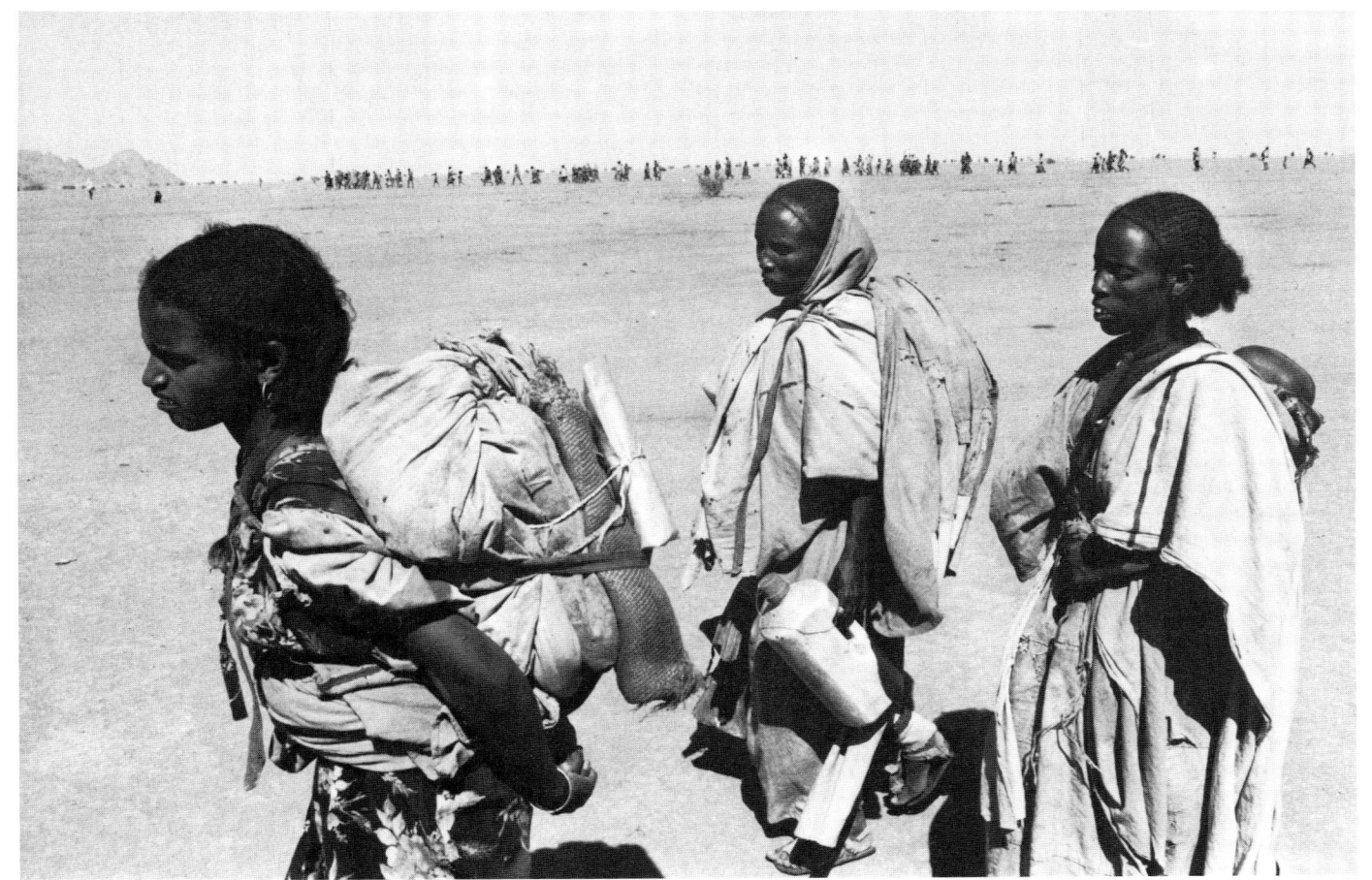

FROM ONE DISASTER TO ANOTHER

Tigrayans arriving at Tukulabab refugee camp in eastern Sudan. Many had walked for six weeks to get here.

Sudan has been host to refugees from Eritrea for more than 20 years, and more recently to people from Tigray. The bulk of the refugee population arrived having fled civil wars in their own provinces. By autumn of 1984, refugees in Sudan already numbered three quarters of a million, most of them settled in camps in the eastern region or in the northern towns. But from October onwards, weary Tigrayans began moving over the border into Sudan in groups which often numbered several thousand. They reported that the Ethiopian government was withholding food relief from civilians in the rebel-held areas.

Faced with starvation in their villages, or resettlement by often hostile troops in other parts of Ethiopia, many of the worst-affected Tigrayan peasants saw no option but to pick up their few meagre possessions and begin the long trek into Sudan. Many arrived after journeys through the mountains of the central region of up to six weeks. They were succoured on their journey by the Relief Society of Tigray, the humanitarian counterpart of the Tigrayan Peoples' Liberation Front, who provided sorghum flour and basic medical supplies at rest stops along the route. On arrival in Sudan the drought refugees came to rest at several different points just inside the border. At one, Tukulubab, the site itself offered no relief whatsoever. In a barren dusty plain within sight of the mountains of Ethiopia, the refugees crouched under thorn bushes for shade by day and huddled to the rocks at night for warmth.

A large-scale relief operation ground into gear, led mainly by the Relief Society of Tigray but with major contributions from the United Nations and from European and American NGOs. But the question which soon arose was how to assist the people to get back to their land in time for the rainy season. Unless the Tigrayans return to get seeds into the ground they condemn them-selves to the prospect of lives of dependency on emergency aid, in refugee camps which are miserably overcrowded. Migrating to Sudan may then appear to have been a disastrous choice for these people, who now number more than 200,000. If more relief agencies had been prepared to attempt to get food aid into Tigray, the poorest people would not have been faced with a choice between starving in their villages or migrating to famine-stricken Sudan.

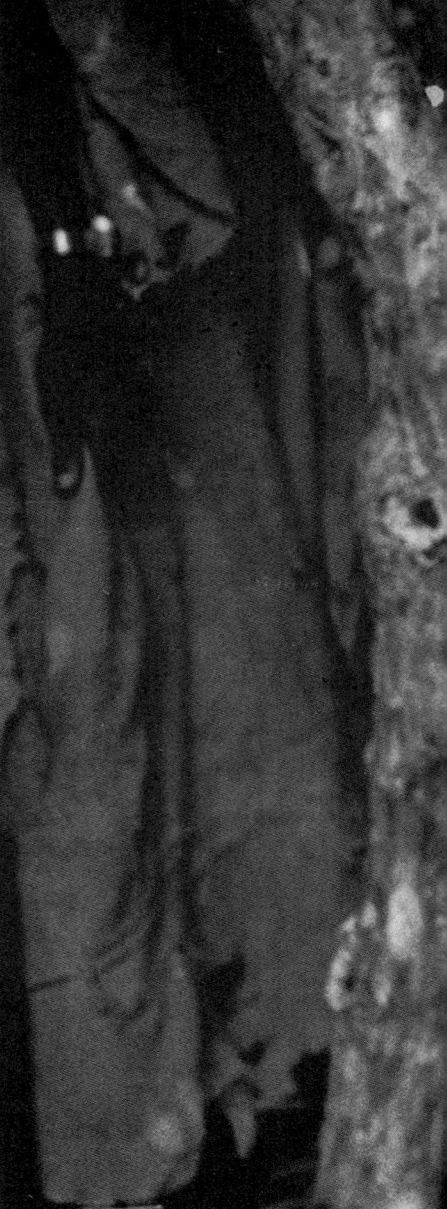

A boy helps a child to a feeding centre in Wad Kowli camp.

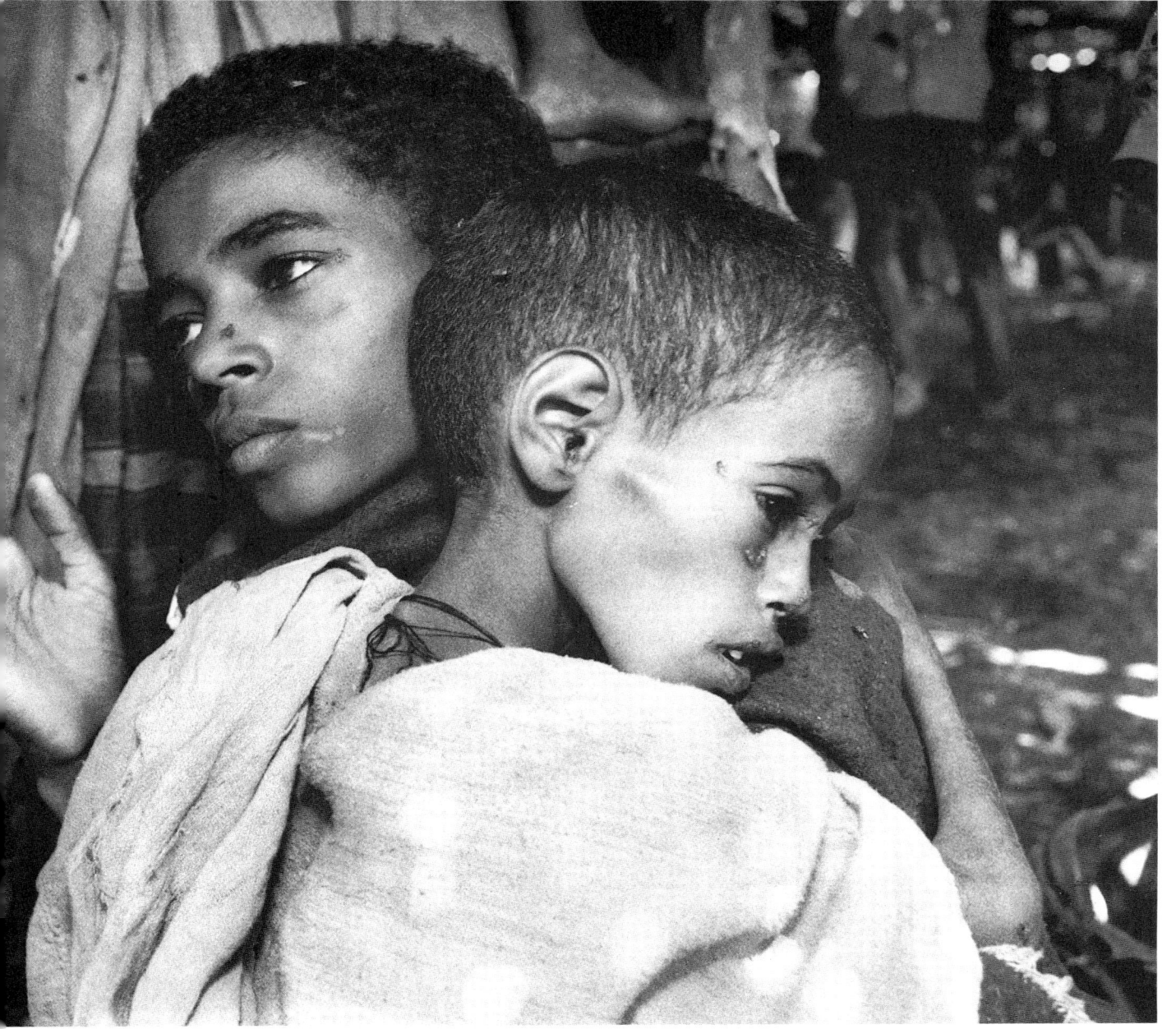

58

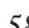

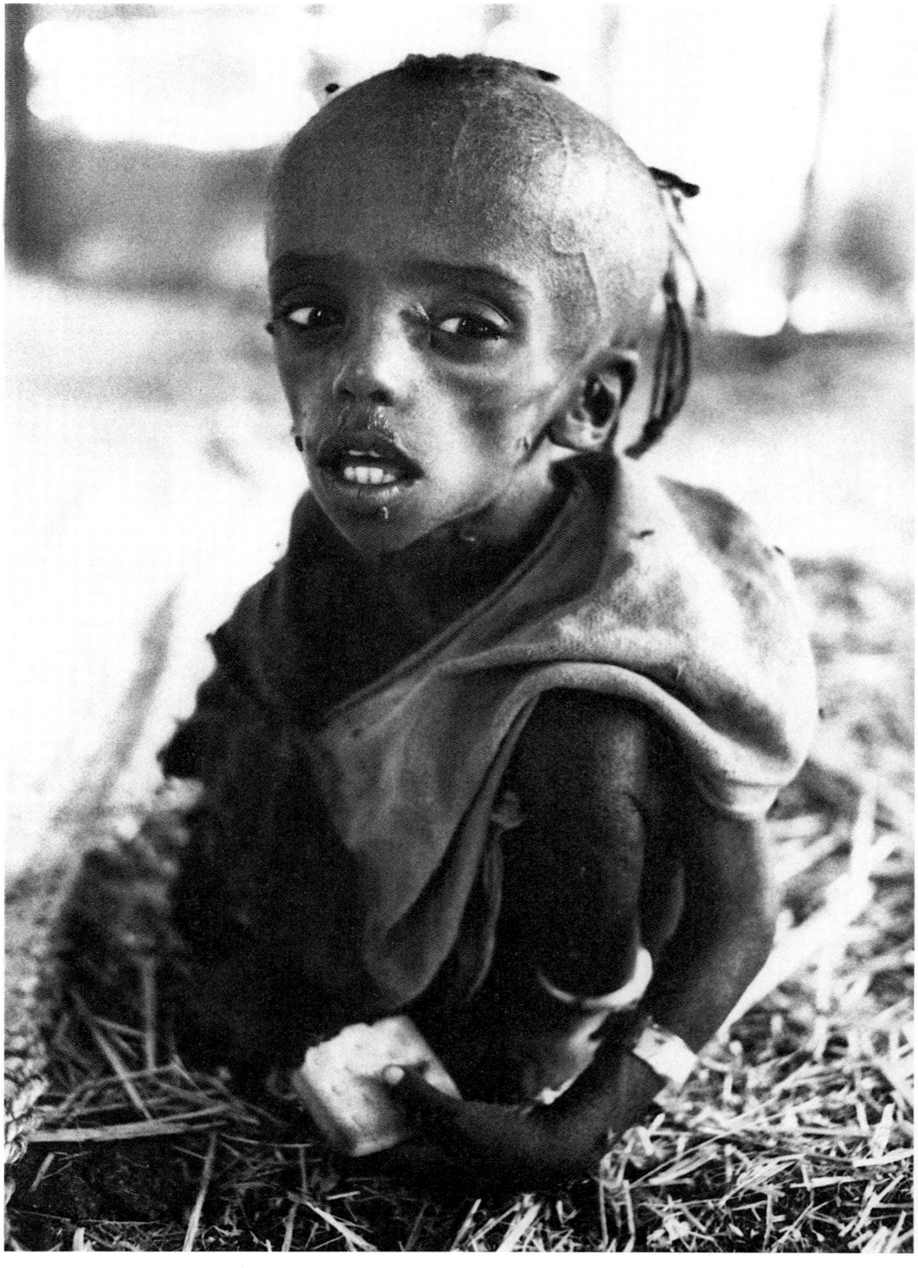

A child in the camp hospital at Wad Kowli.

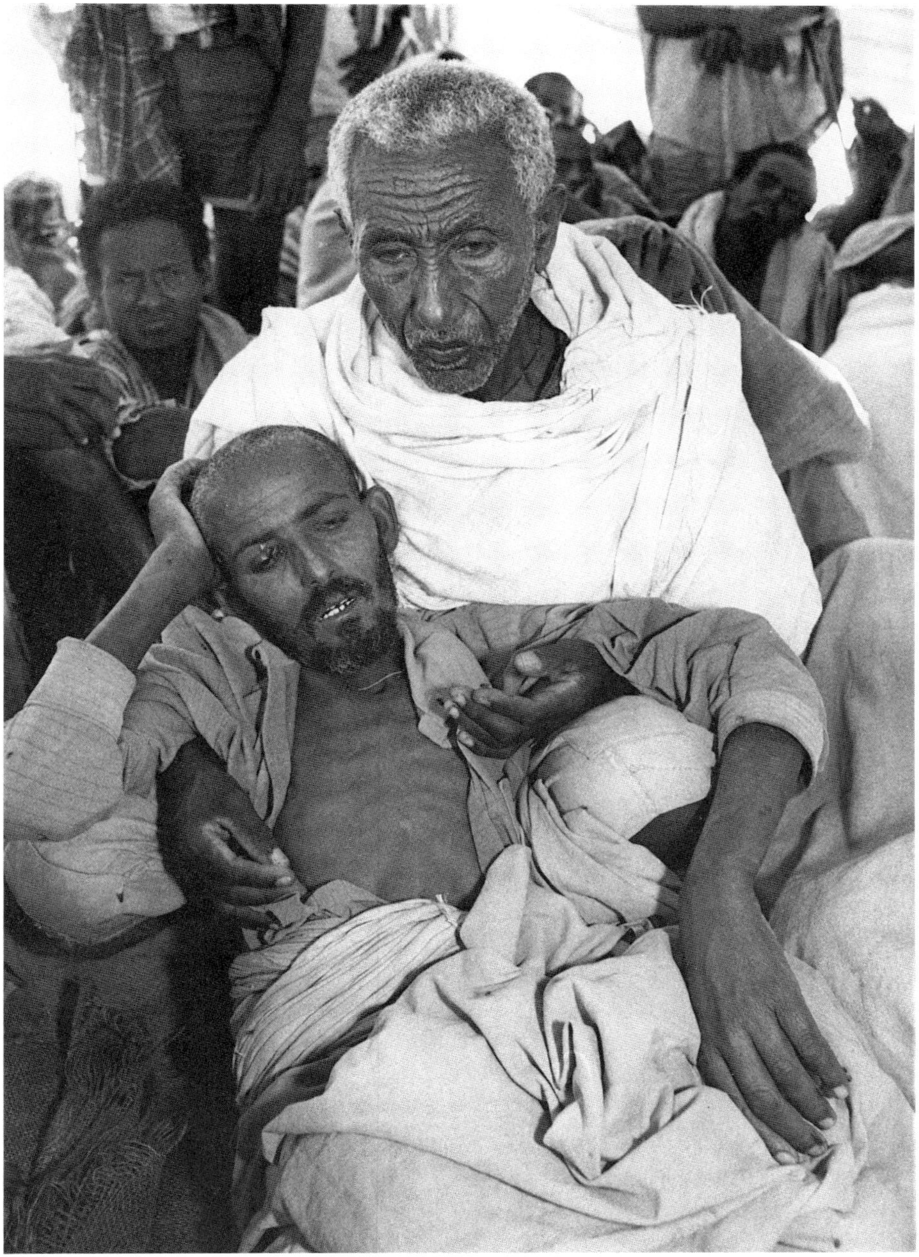

59

A father cares for his son in Tukulabab camp.

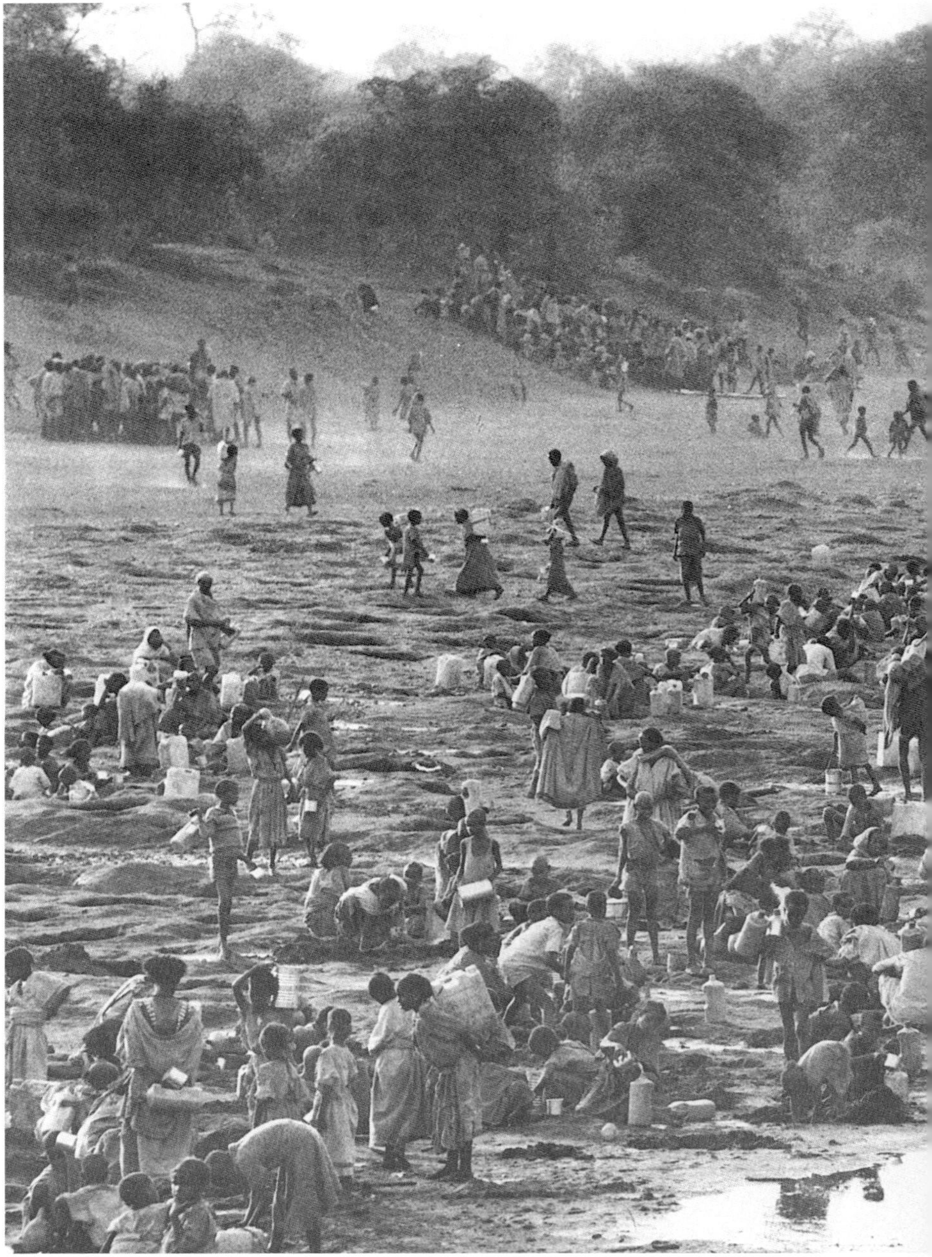

60

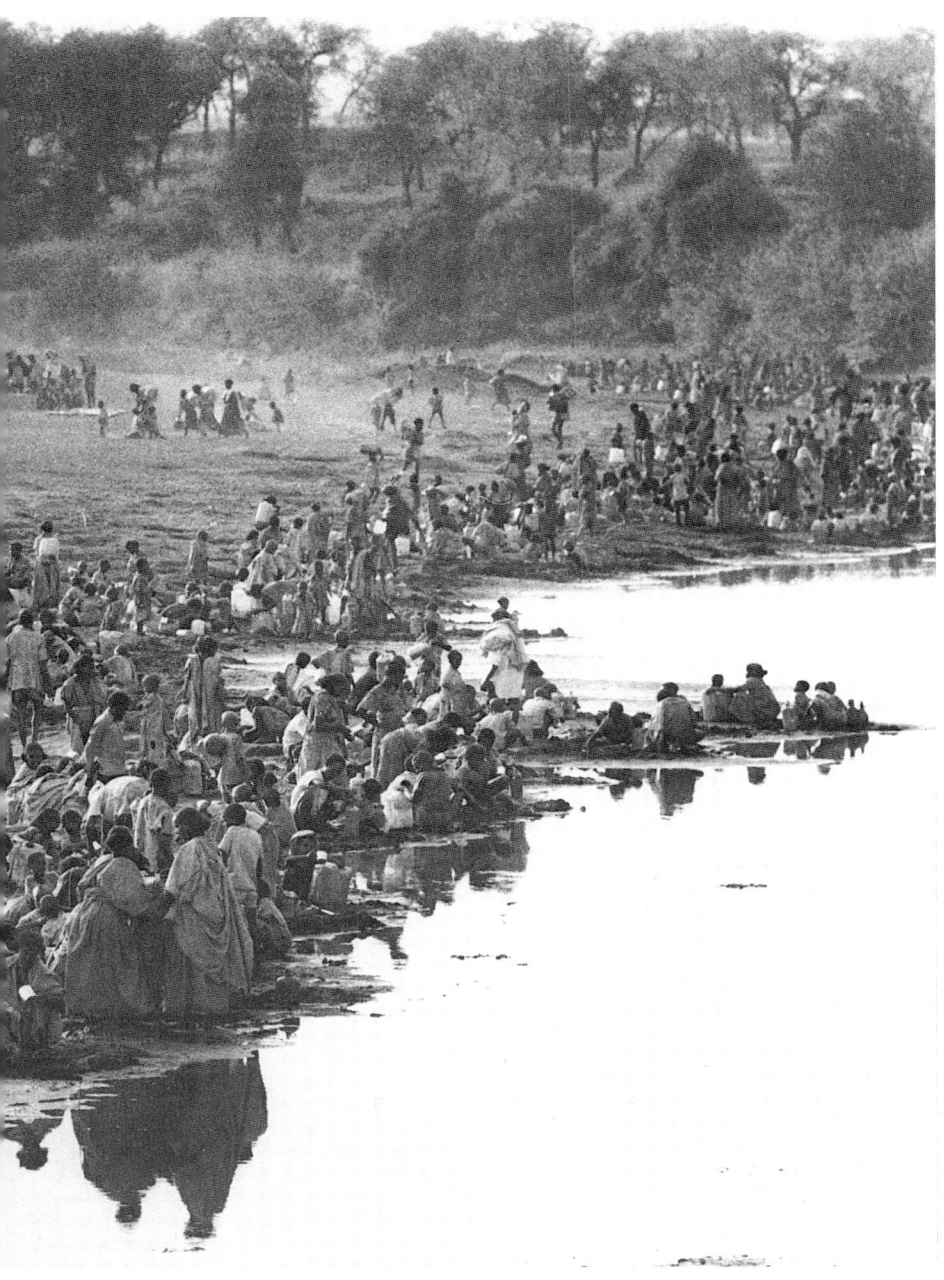

Once the northern route out of Tigray had been closed at the border by the Sudanese authorities, people fleeing the drought began to arrive at Wad Kowli, a camp further south, close to the border at Gedaref. By the end of January, 100,000 Tigrayans had gathered here. Aid agencies constructed hospitals to treat the sick and set up feeding centres for the malnourished, but the camp was hopelessly overcrowded. The river, the only source of water, dwindled daily.

61

In mid-January, 100 people per day were dying in Wad Kowli, although within a few weeks the efforts of relief workers helped to reduce the death rate by half.

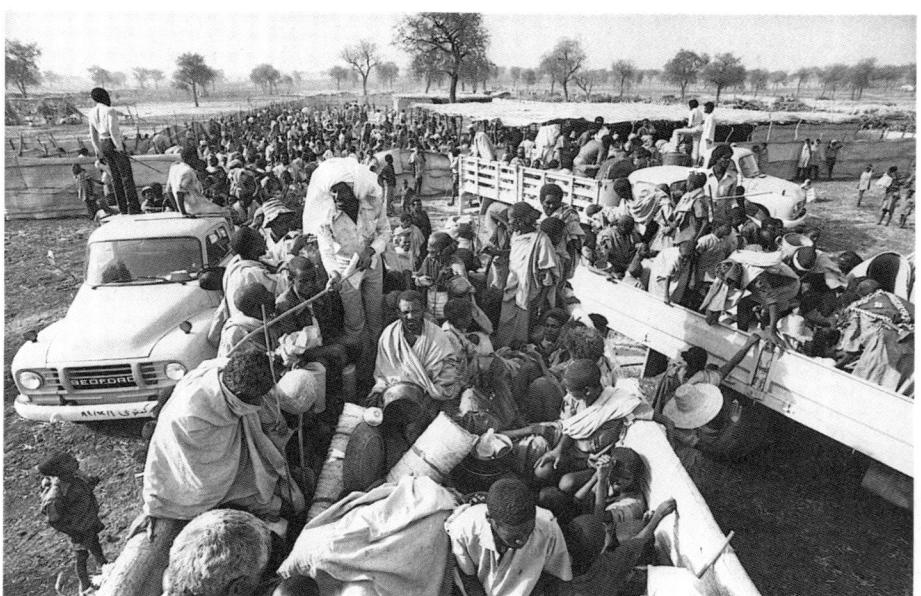

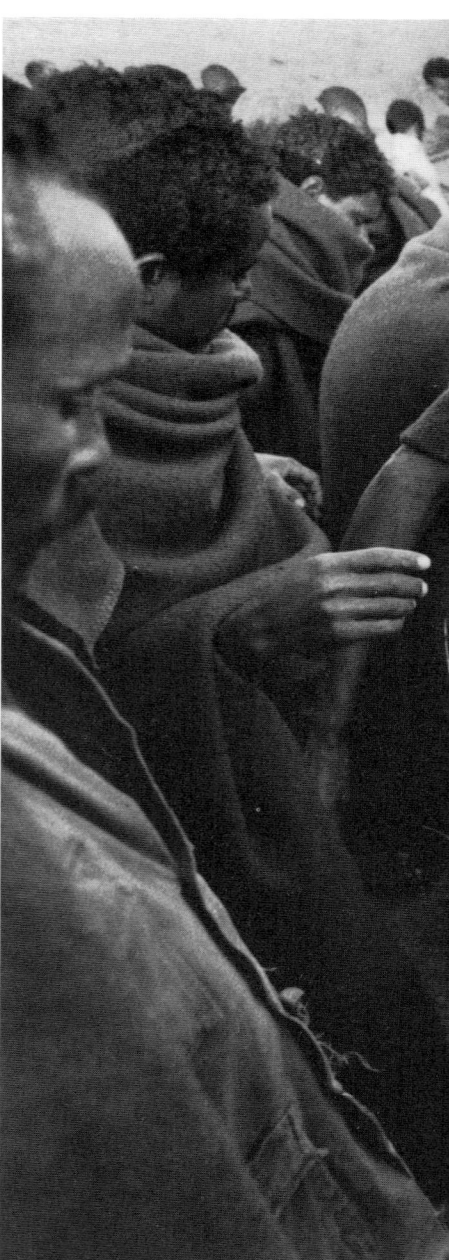

In an attempt to lessen the overcrowding and the pressure on the meagre water supplies, the Sudanese refugee authority began moving people from Wad Kowli to another camp at Safawa, two hours' drive away. Shortages of fuel and trucks meant that a maximum of 2,000 people could be moved daily. Meanwhile, more Tigrayan refugees were arriving.

62

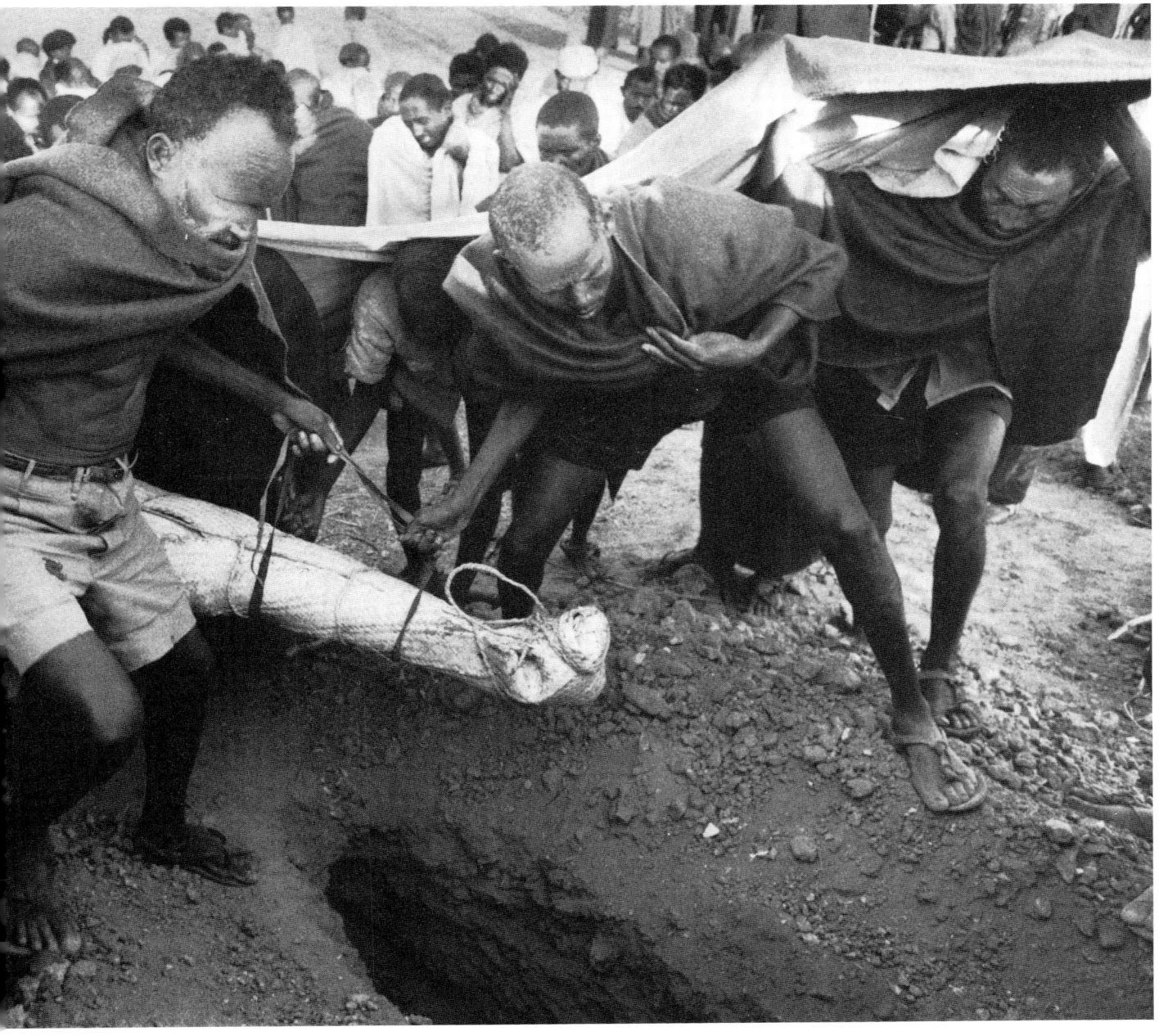

63

Despite these pressures, more than three million people have remained in Tigray. Markets are full of people trying to sell anything from donkeys to woven shawls, but buyers are few and far between. Many people have nothing left to sell. They have eaten the seed grain meant for planting this year, sold the animals with which they would have ploughed the land, and gone heavily into debt in order to buy food.

United Nations and bilateral aid continues to be channelled through the Ethiopian government, despite the fact that much of rural Tigray is now controlled by the Tigrayan Peoples' Liberation Front (TPLF), who are leading a liberation struggle in the province against the Ethiopian government. Ironically, it is in this small war-torn province in Ethiopia – which has received virtually no outside assistance for a decade – that some of the potentially most workable examples of development programmes are to be found.

Agriculture is the livelihood of over 90 per cent of the people of Tigray, most of whom grow little more food than they need to survive, even in normal times. The major threat to agricultural improvement, as in so much of Africa, is soil erosion. Within Tigray, rainfall has almost always been sufficient for farmers to produce enough food. But centuries of land misuse, combined with negligible technological development, have produced acute rural poverty. Surpluses were siphoned off in taxes by the feudal landlords during the Selassie dynasty, and little capital re-invested in the rural infrastructure. Sixty per cent of the rural population live in the central region of Tigray and, as the land became gradually poorer, all land that could possibly be cultivated was brought under the plough. This included much steeply sloping land from which virtually all the original forest cover had been removed. Shrub and grass cover decreased, and flash floods rushed down the denuded escarpments taking the topsoil with them. A recent survey revealed that each year 17 tonnes of topsoil are being eroded per single hectare of land in the central highlands.

In response to the famine, the Ethiopian government has been moving people out of the areas it still controls and resettling them in other parts of the country, on the grounds that Tigray's exhausted soil can no longer support the population. An unstated second reason exists for such a strategy – by dispersing the population of the rebel province the government hopes to undermine the movement fighting for self-determination.

Abi Adi in central Tigray on market day. Thousands of people come in from the outlying villages, but the drought has left resources low and there are many more sellers than buyers.

64

Tigray

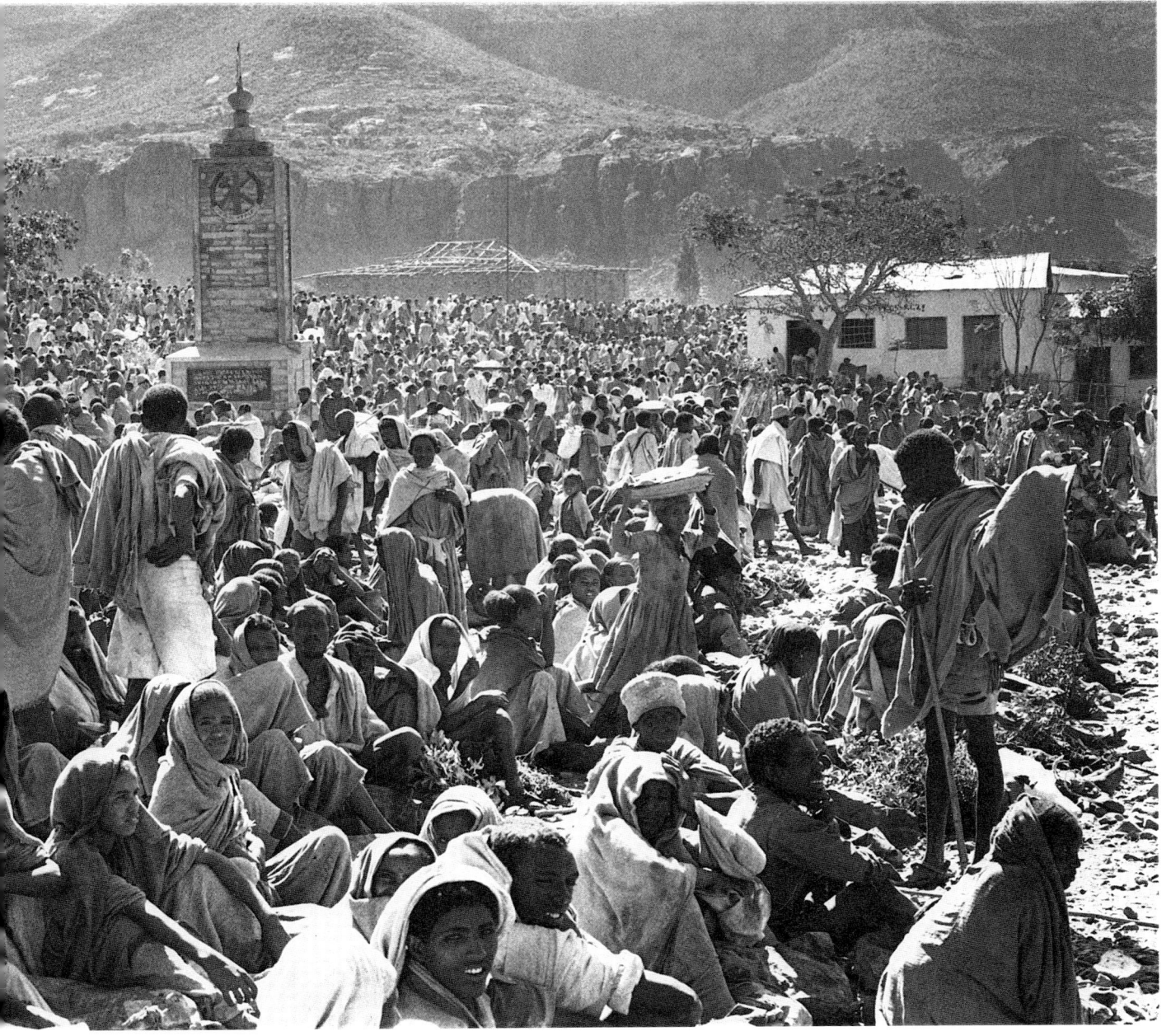

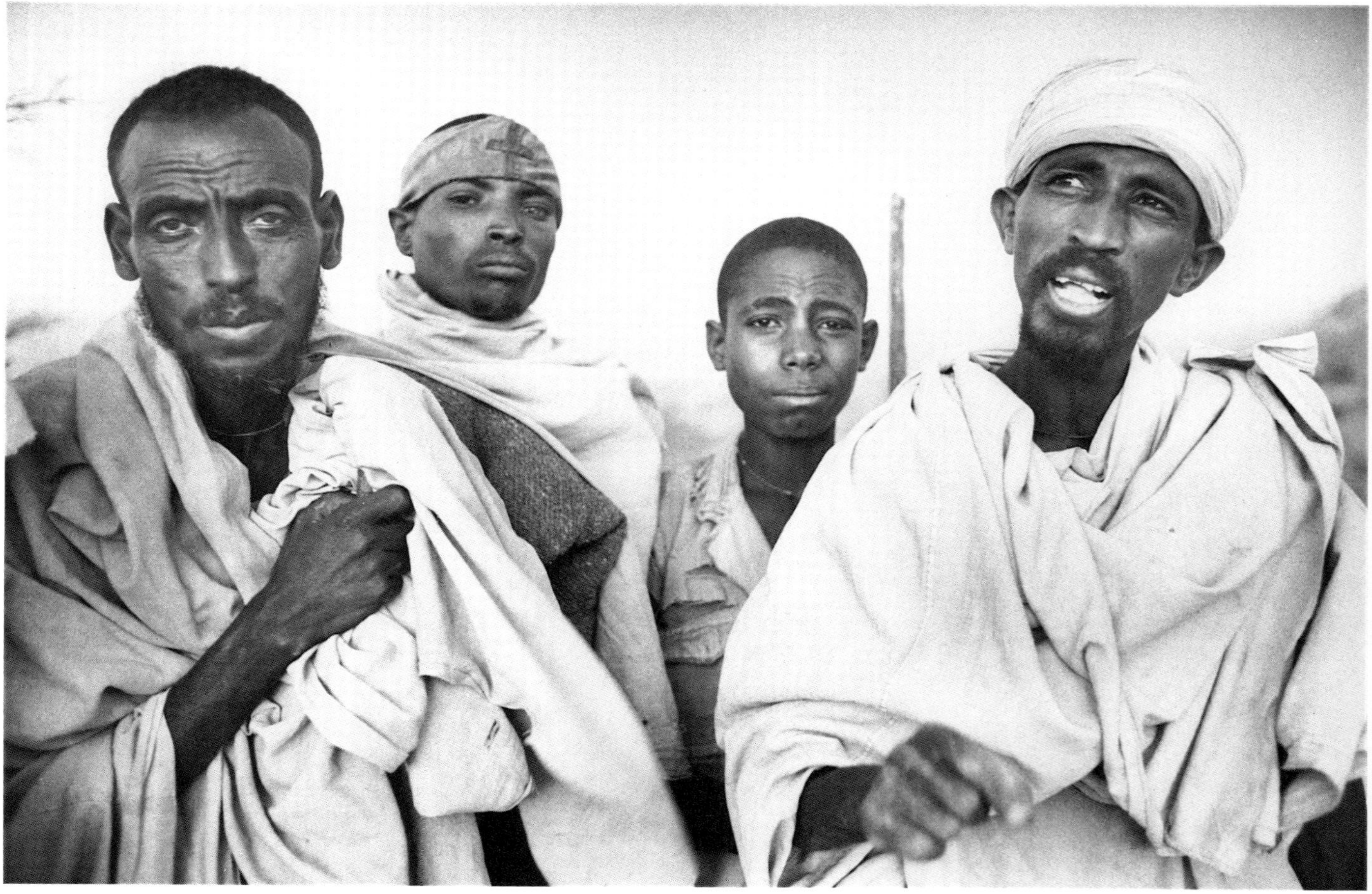

66

'The Ethiopian soldiers surrounded our village [near Axum, northern Tigray] and said we had to go for resettlement. We had enough food and some money so we refused to go. But they took us by force. At Axum we were made to get on an aeroplane to Makelle. We went to see the administrator there to try and get home, but he refused to listen to us. People who would not get on the plane to Addis were beaten with sticks and one was killed. We were flown to Addis. When we arrived at the airport there were buses waiting to take us to Jima. We arrived at the reception centre in the dark. We could not wait to escape. We asked if we could go outside to urinate, and then ran to cross the river. We walked all night and slept in the forest. We got lost but eventually we found a route north. It took us a month to walk back here [to Finarawa in Tigray]. We are going back to our villages now. We don't know whether our families are still there or not.'

Gabre Mikhel Sium (priest)

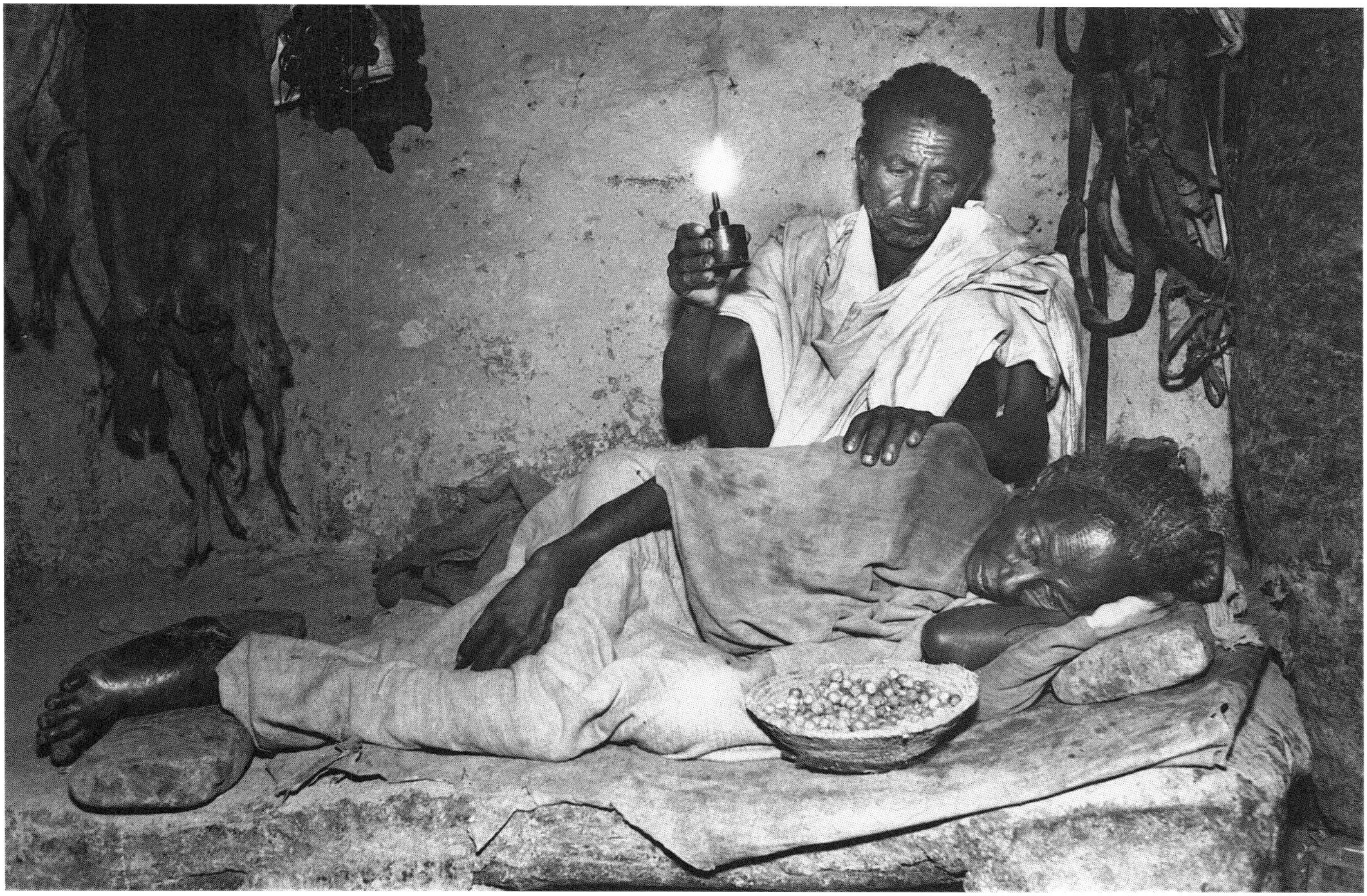

'I went to Sudan five months ago from my village [near Samre, central Tigray] and came back bringing two watches and some money I had earned working in fields in Sudan. On the way back, at Abderafi, the garrison town, Ethiopian militia men stole all the money. But I had the watches stuffed down my trousers. While I was away my mother-in-law here, Saubatu Abio, went to the city of Makelle to get food. She went to the feeding camp, but they wouldn't give her anything. She survived by begging and two weeks later some relatives brought her back by mule. But now she is sick. We have no grain left, and we are eating our cattle to survive. I had three cows and one ox. The ox was sold while I was in Sudan. We still have meat from the last of the cows which we slaughtered today. I have sold the two watches and so I have a little money, and I still have one donkey. I will go to Belesa to buy grain. It is a four-day walk. The donkey can carry half a quintel (50 kilos) which will cost me 50 Birr (Ethiopian dollars). I will sell half in Abi Adi for about 40 Birr. The other half we will live on. It will keep us going for two weeks.'

Teferse Gabrezedcon

Agriculture

The Tigrayans are unwilling to leave their lands. They have been making efforts to improve agricultural techniques, and to develop soil and water conservation methods which relieve the pressure on the land. Their first major soil conservation project was at Showata, a steeply sloped area in the lowlands on the sheltered side of the Semien mountains. It is in the very centre of the drought-stricken area. Twenty hectares were successfully terraced for irrigation by using a 450-metre long main canal with a series of feeder canals and terrace bands.

It took 32,000 'person days' to complete the work, according to the Tigrayan Peoples' Liberation Front who organized the project. But it paid off. Technically, the scheme is a huge success, yielding two harvests a year in an area where no other farms are producing anything in the current drought. The Showata project demonstrates the possibilities for agriculture in capturing and controlling rainfall. But its operation requires specific engineering skills which few Tigrayans have, and skilled people need to be permanently on site to oversee and maintain the system. Such a scheme cannot be adopted by the mass of the population on their individual fields. The Relief Society of Tigray (REST) has trained 2,000 peasants so far in an alternative 'water spreading' technique which requires only elementary training and a simple spirit level. Similar techniques have been developed elsewhere in Africa, but governments have rarely given priority to such 'appropriate technology'. The programme includes methods for levelling fields and terracing slopes with stone walls to contain the rainfall. Only mass participation will have any significant effect in halting soil erosion, and REST hopes to use the trained farmers to spread the techniques in their villages.

Dwindling harvests over the last few years, caused by drought, have meant that participants in the Tigrayan conservation schemes have had to be supplied with food for their work, mainly to provide them with enough energy to do these taxing physical activities. But experience with 'food for work' programmes elsewhere in Africa shows them to be largely negative in effect, as summed up by a report on a similar anti-erosion scheme in Burkina Faso in 1980, which commented that 'the use of food aid as an incentive to farmers to participate in community development programmes has distorted their conception of the value of the work, and undermined the interest that a farmer usually has in the future of his community. Among farmers who have received food aid in the past for community development work, the overriding concern is with the food aid'.

In short, people were persuaded to participate in 'community development' projects because they wanted the food, not because they were committed to the value of the work they were doing. One implication is that maintenance will not be continued, a problem which has arisen with collective tree-planting schemes in Mali. People were paid in food to plant the trees and now nobody is prepared to look after them, unless they are paid with more food.

Self-reliance

But the Tigrayan context is somewhat different. The population has grown into the habit of self-reliance, as a result of the continued strife and relative isolation in which they live. Food aid here seems to function as a necessary support to an initiative to which people are already committed, rather than as a means of enticing people into doing something in which they were not previously interested.

Changing conditions have also affected the lives of women in Tigray. So many Tigrayan men have joined the TPLF army, or been killed in the war, or have left for the Sudan, that there has been a desperate need for women to step outside their traditional roles as unpaid labourers on their husbands' fields, with the backbreaking tasks of weeding the crops by hand and harvesting by sickle. Much of the drudgery of women's lives remains. Women still do the hardest and most menial work such as fetching water and pounding grain into flour. Nonetheless, their position has improved. Previously, girls could be married at ages as young as nine years, in arrangements which had contractual advantages for the families involved. Now they have won the right to choose their own husbands and to initiate divorce proceedings.

Necessity has prompted their moving into a whole range of other activities which were previously the exclusive preserve of men. As well as sharing responsibility for farming, from ploughing to harvesting, women now hold 30 per cent of the elected positions on the Peoples' Councils around the province, and constitute the majority of the judiciary. The rapidly changing position of women is an interesting indication of the development of Tigrayan society as a whole.

Most recently, the Tigrayans have undertaken their own operation in response to the drought. The only way to get emergency food aid from Sudan to the worst-hit parts of the country has been to build a road across the gorge which cuts off the west of the province from the central highlands. They have built the road with little more than picks and shovels. If a large rock blocked the path, they lit a fire underneath to crack it. With few qualified engineers, they had to learn about road construction the hard way. Some bends were at first built too sharp, and some slopes too steep. But the road is now complete, and food supplies can be moved to the east, decreasing the numbers of people forced to migrate.

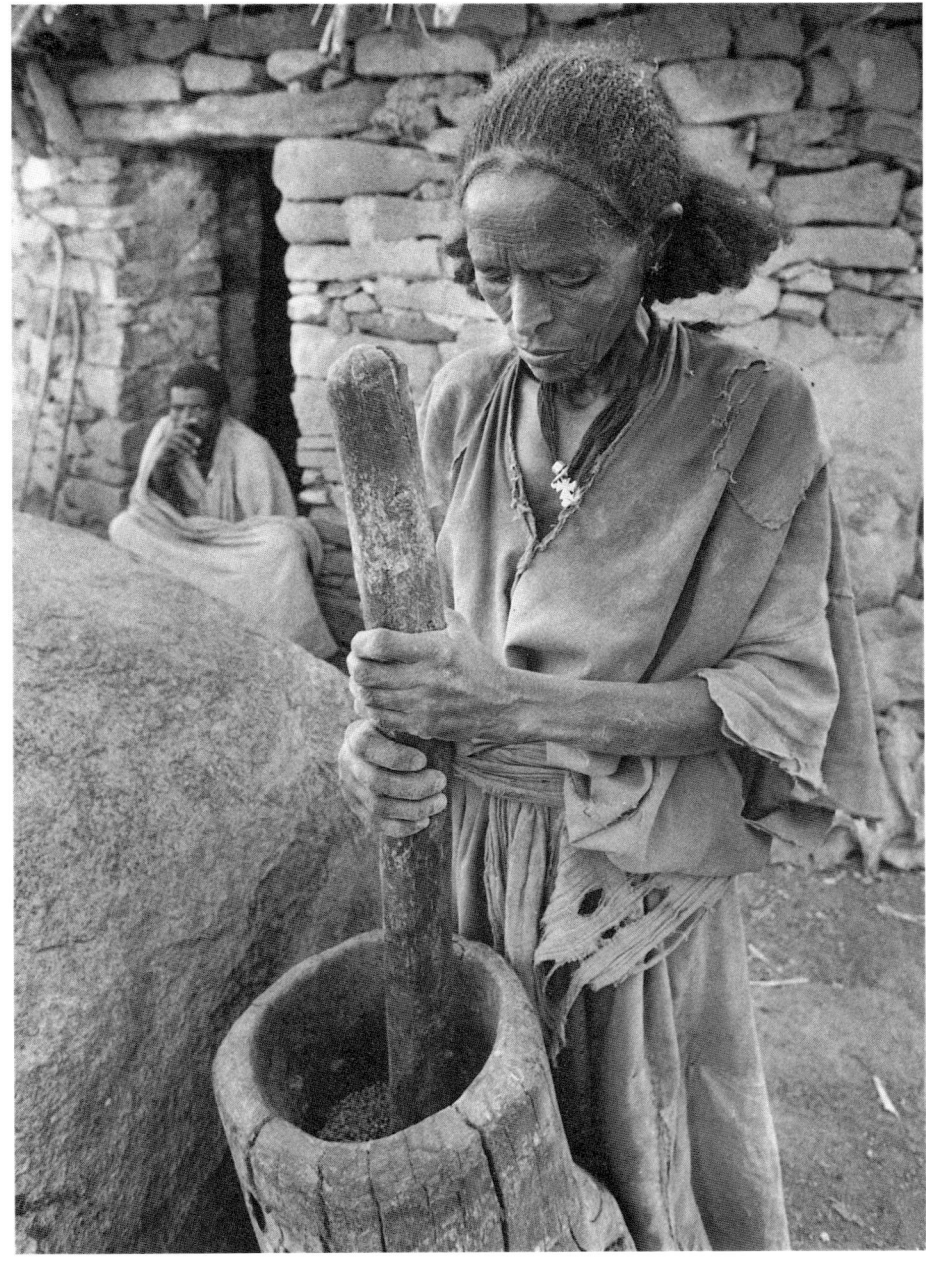

Grain is first pounded, then ground between stones to make flour for injera bread, the Tigrayan staple food. It is always women's work.

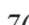

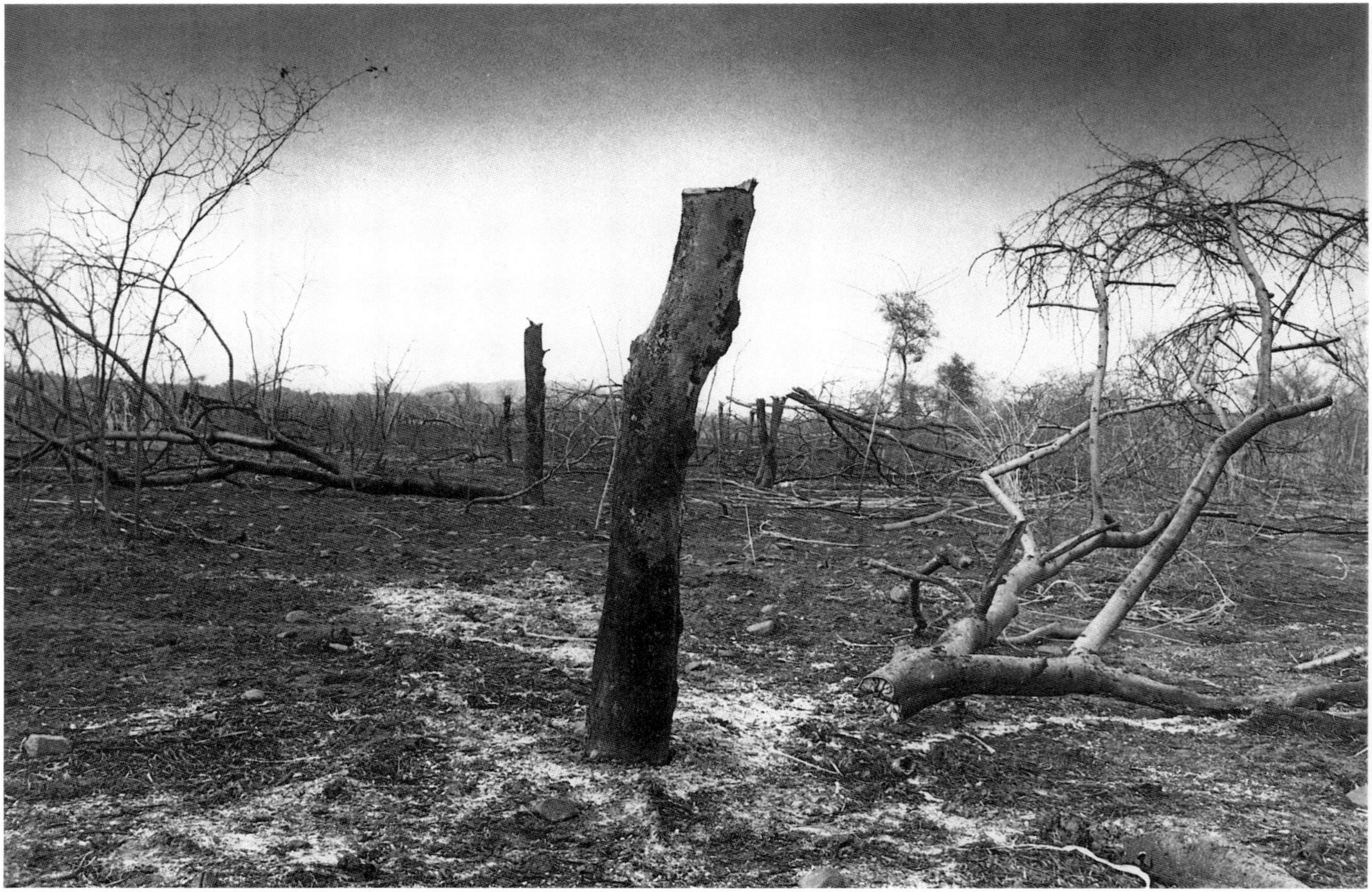

The primary causes of deforestation in
Africa are that land is being cleared for
cultivation by subsistence farmers, and
that trees are being felled for firewood. Soil
erosion is an inevitable consequence.

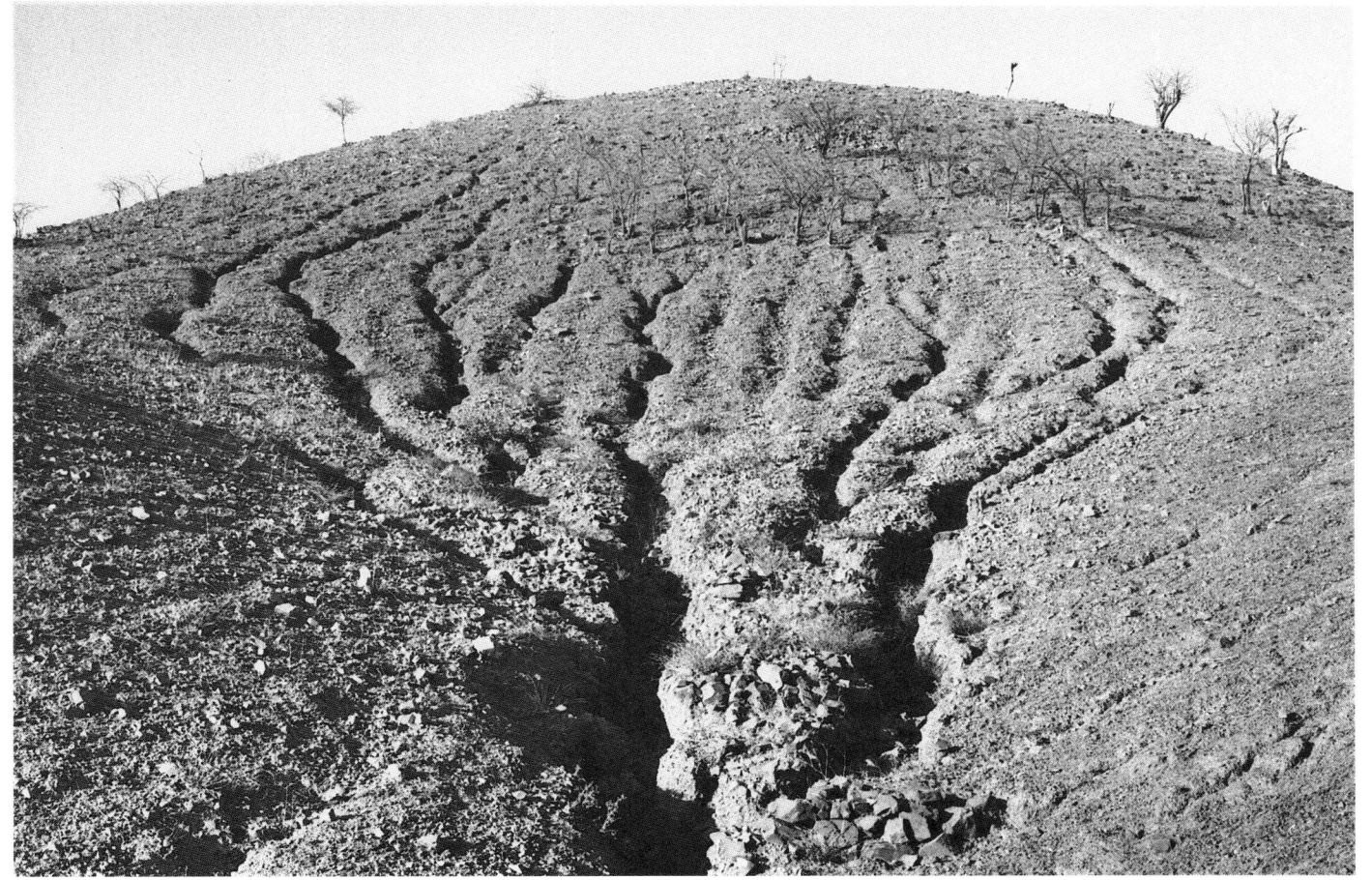

Soil erosion is a natural process as old as the earth itself. But here, in the central region of Tigray, soil erosion following deforestation has increased to the point where it far exceeds the formation of new soil.

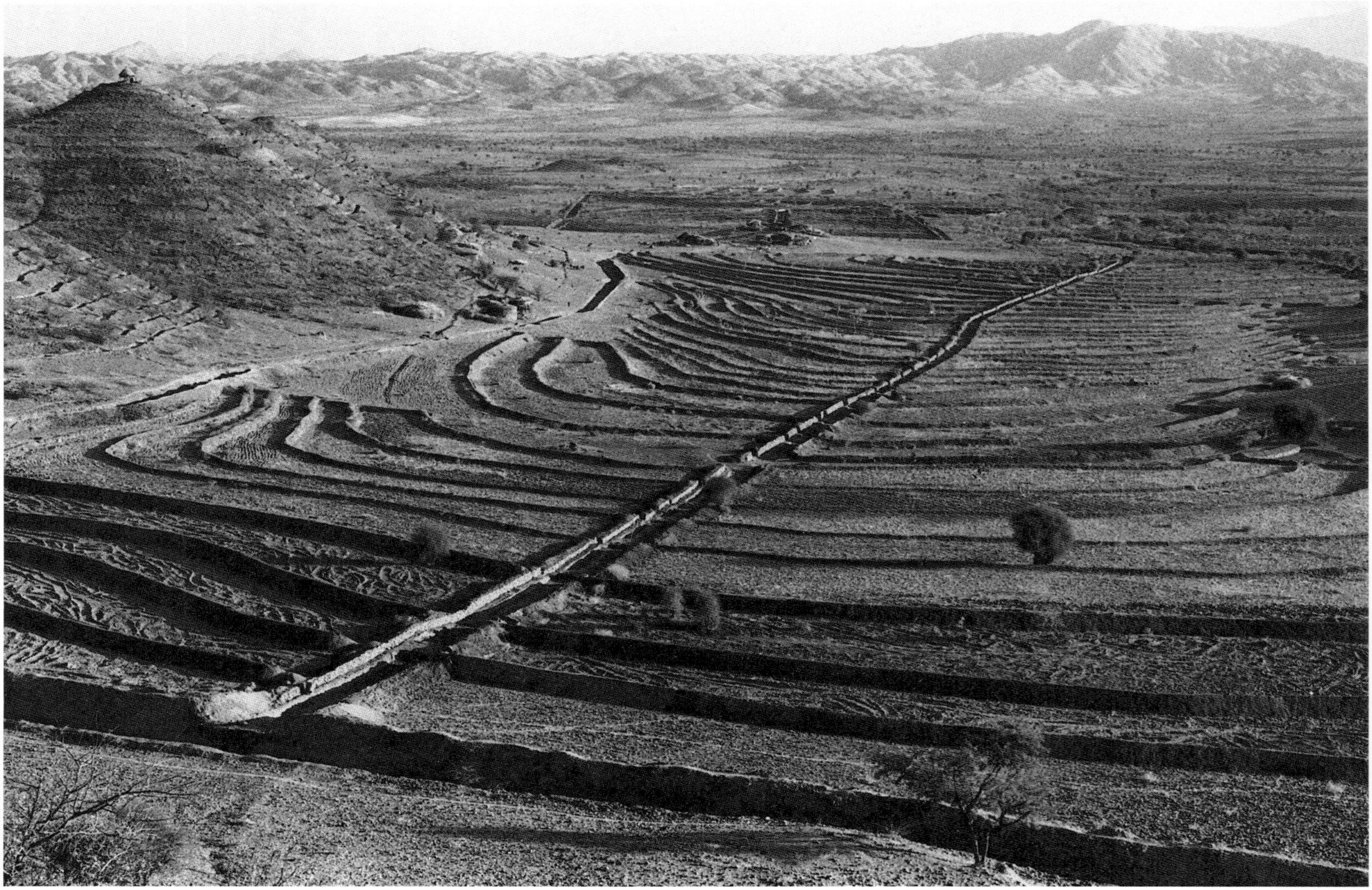

Even in drought years, irrigation schemes
can harness irregular and light rainfalls,
and produce substantial harvests. The
Shawata Project in Central Tigray is in the
middle of the drought area. By chanelling
off part of a nearby river that only flows
after each rain, the irrigated land yields
two good harvests a year.

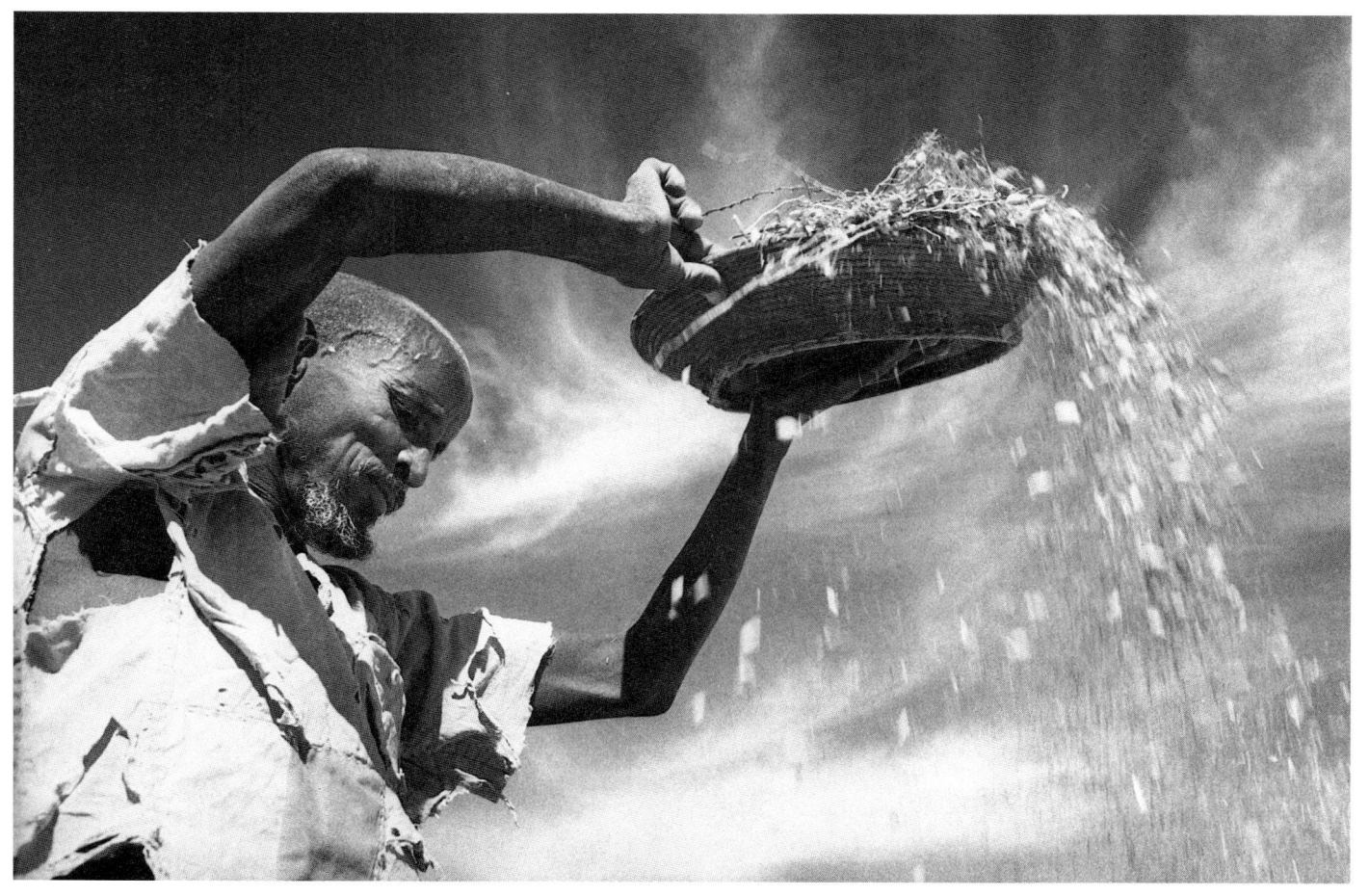

**Winnowing sorghum to separate the grain
from the chaff.**

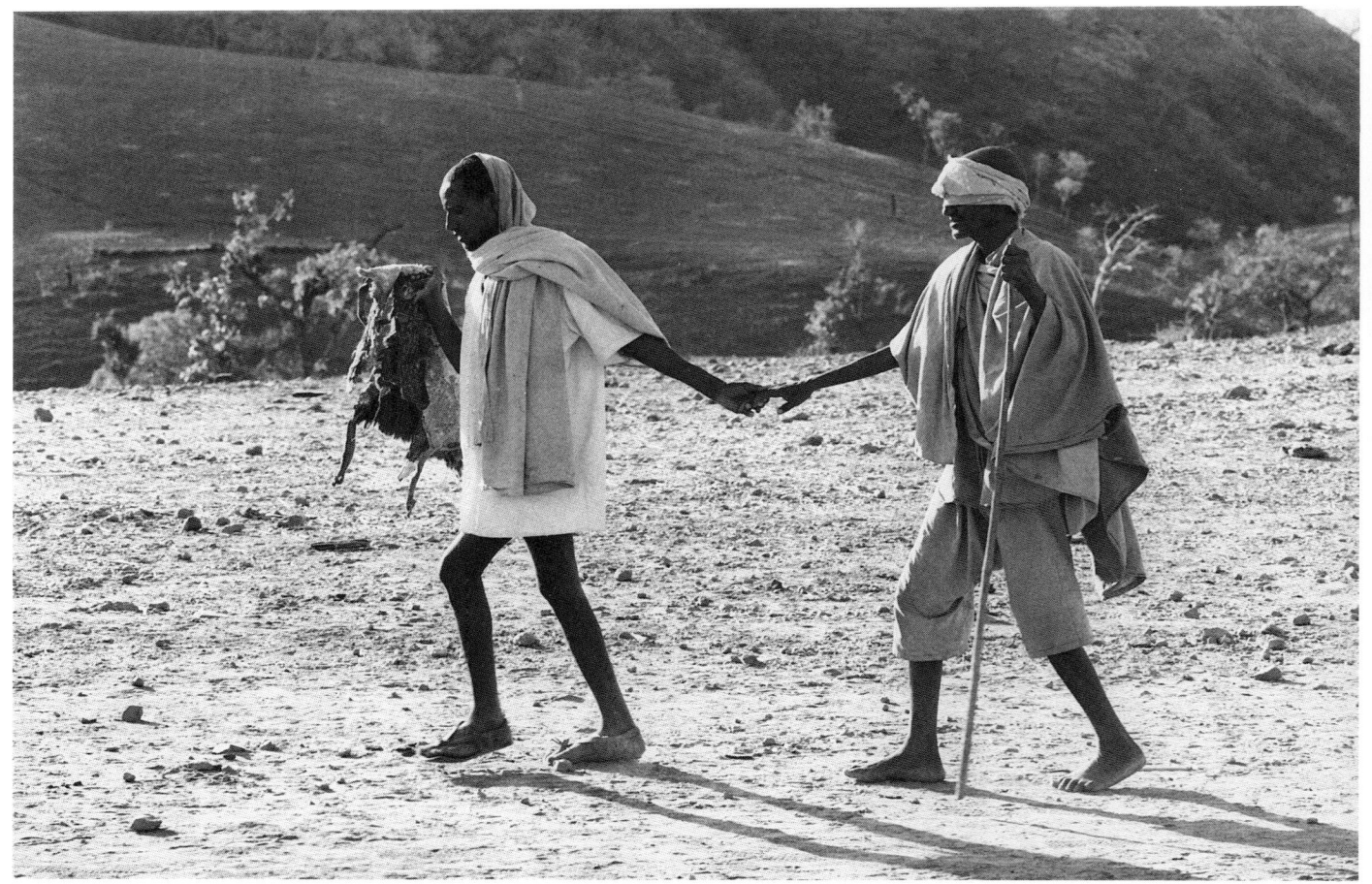

74

Communities have been devastated by the exodus to Sudan.

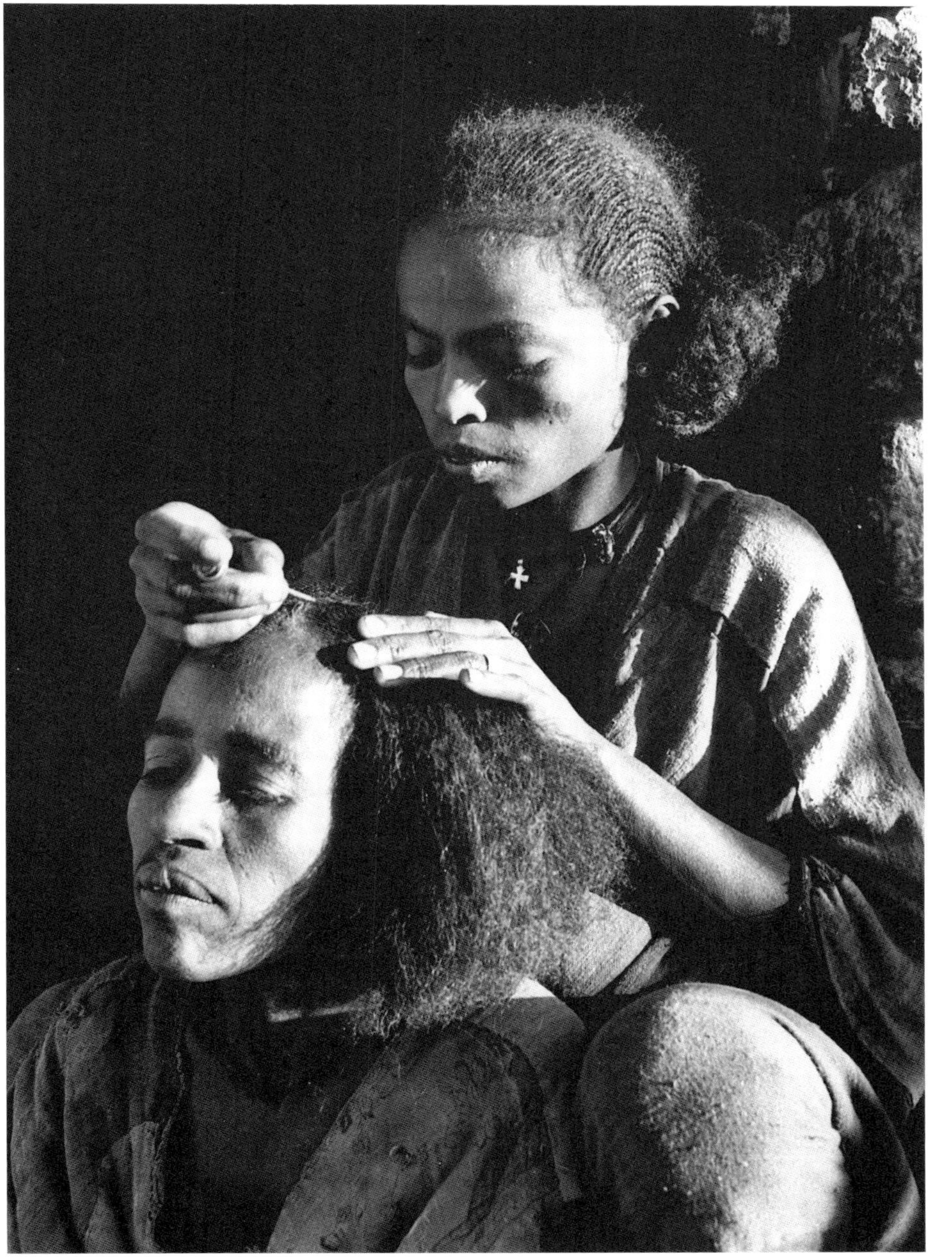

**Plaiting hair. Life carries on for those who
have enough resources to remain in their
villages.**

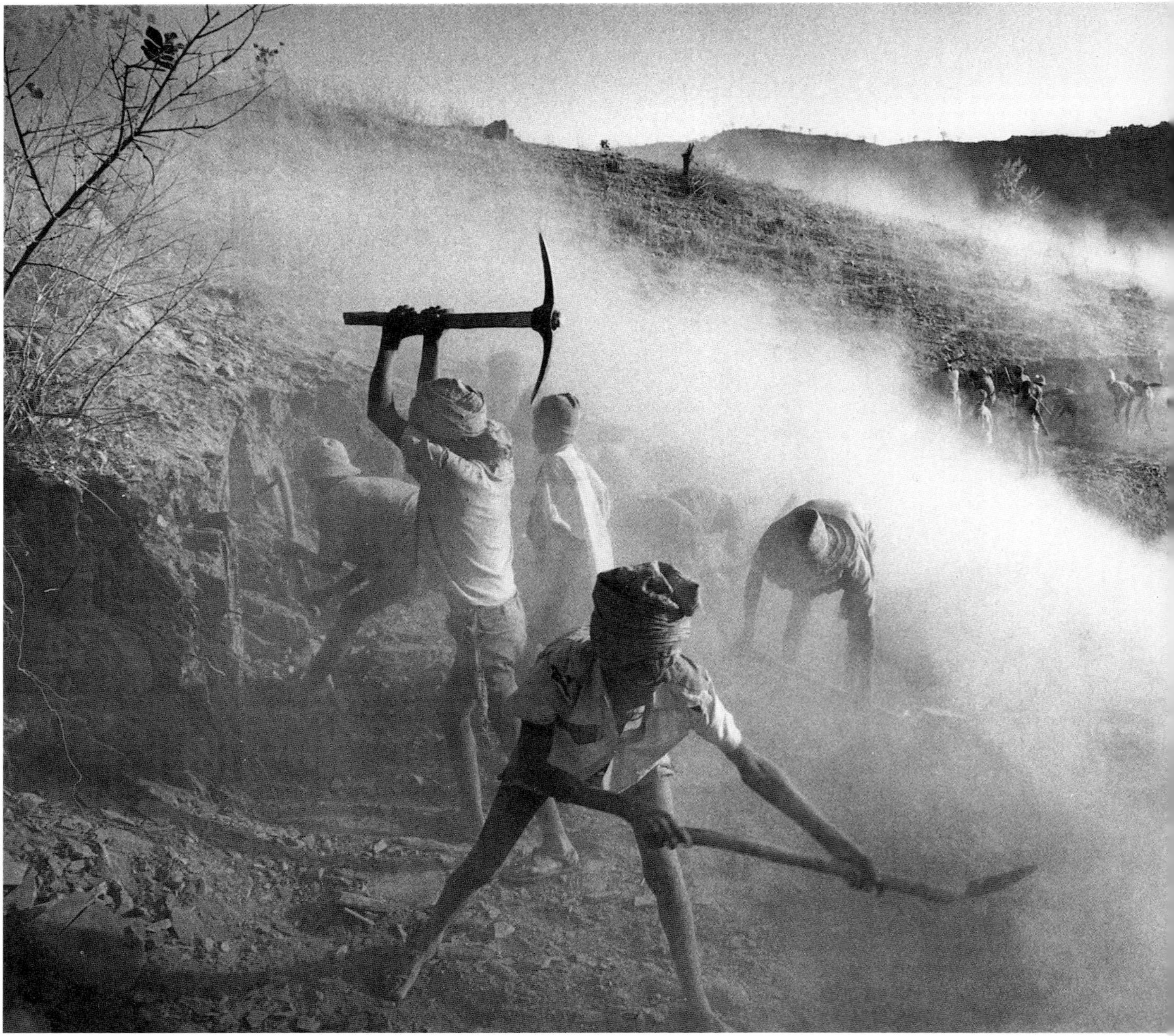

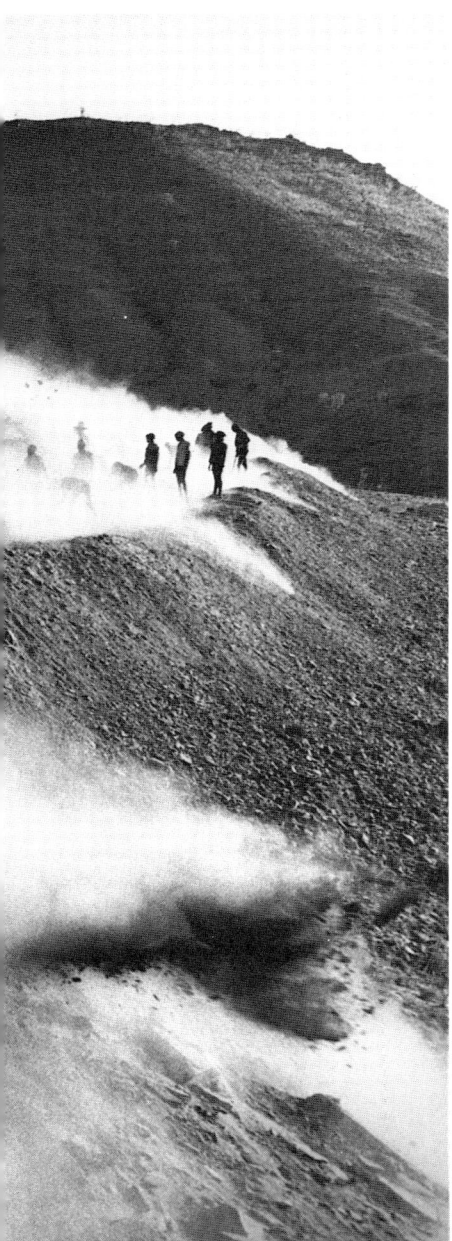

Tigrayans construct a road across the Herme Gorge to link western Tigray with the central region. Until the road was completed in 1985, the only means of transporting food aid to drought-stricken villagers was on the backs of donkeys and camels.

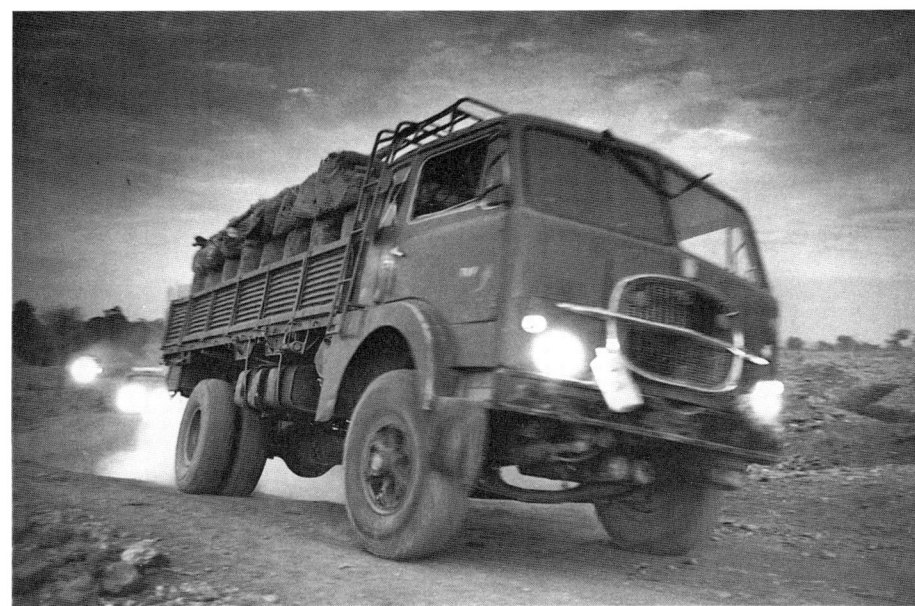

REST brings emergency food into Tigray. Three times a week, convoys of ten trucks make the two-day journey into western Tigray from Kassala in Sudan.

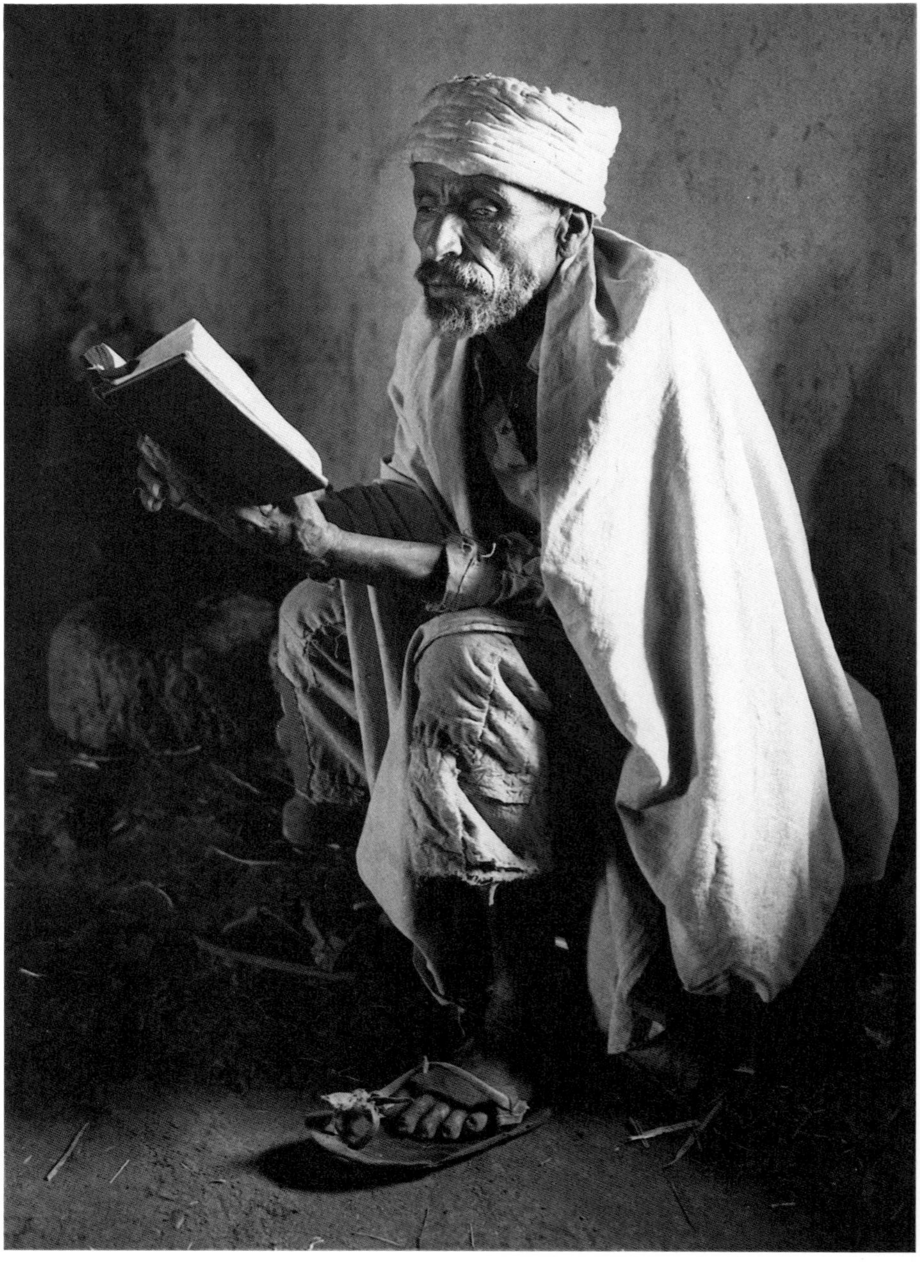

Religion retains a strong hold on Tigrayan society – most of its people are Coptic Christians. This priest reads his bible in Giz, an Ethiopian language dating from the first century AD.

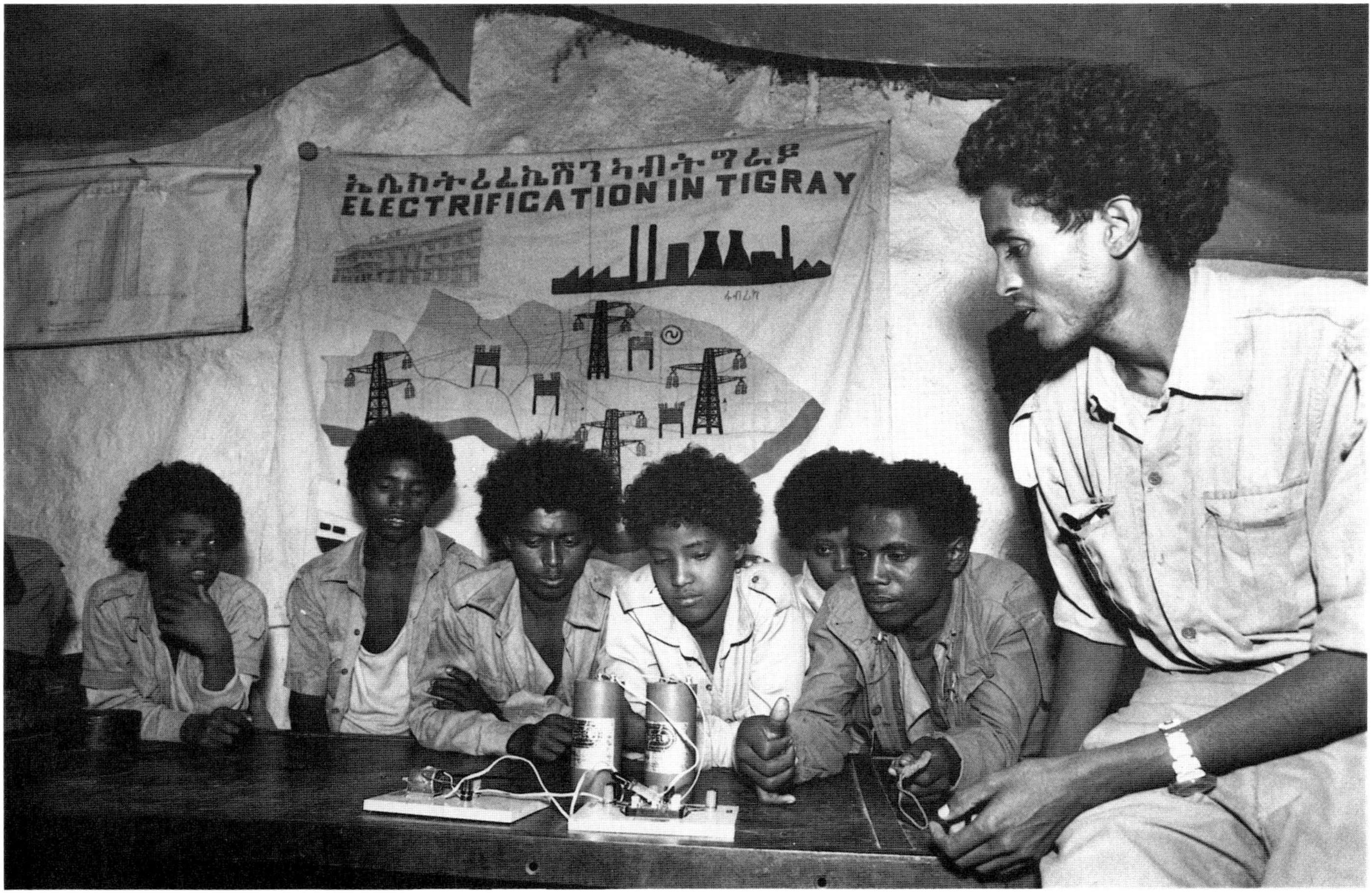

An electrical workshop in Tigray, run by the Tigrayan Peoples' Liberation Front (TPLF). Workshops also teach watch repair, vehicle maintenance, metalwork and radio repair.

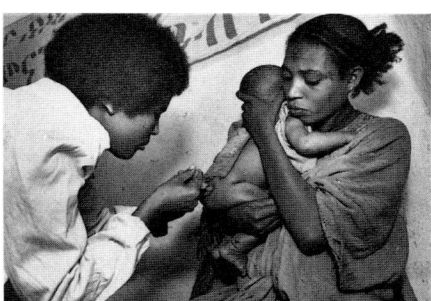

TPLF health centre in Samre, central Tigray.

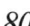

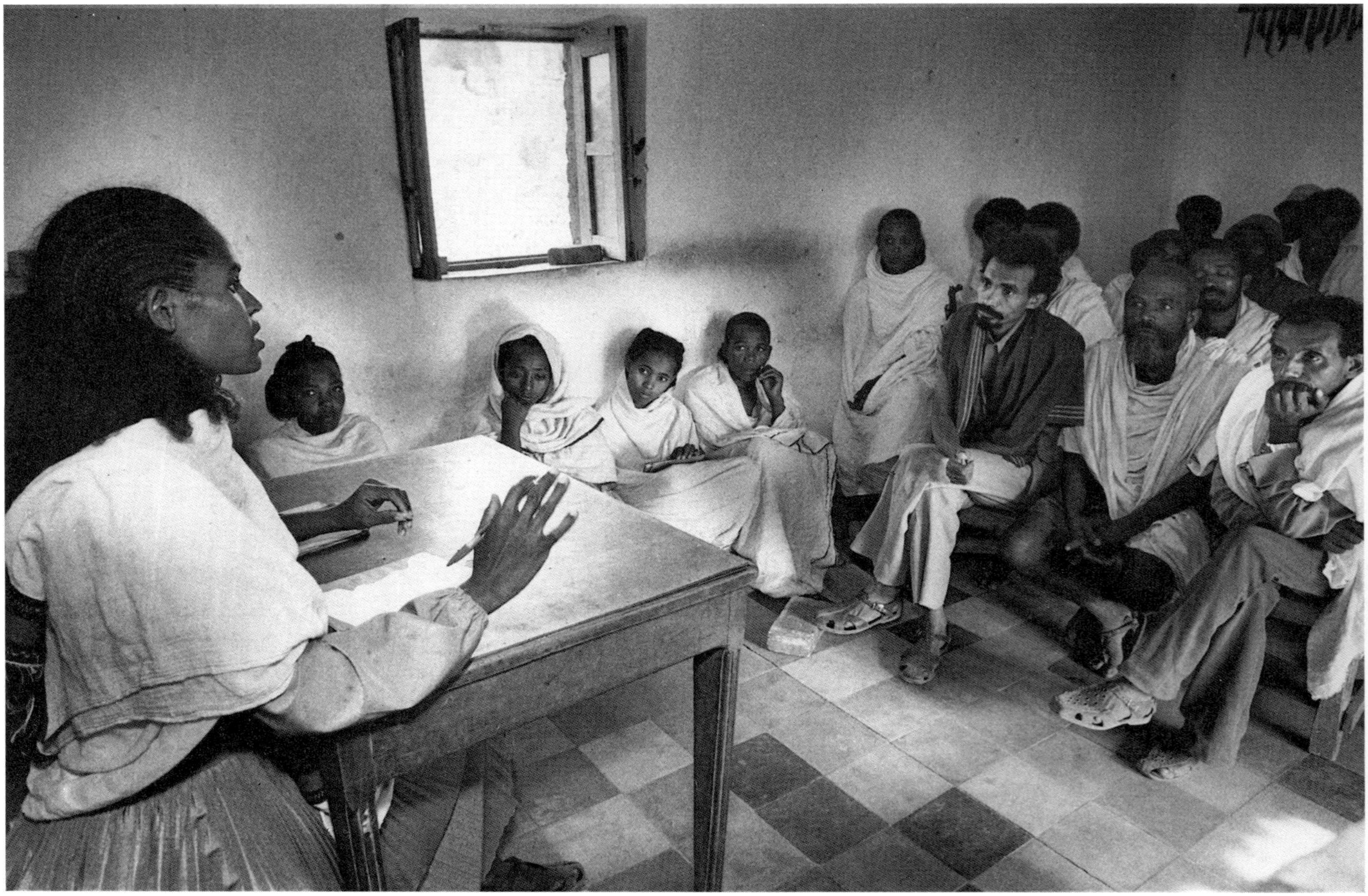

**A woman chairs the 'Bitor' area council
in Abi Adi.**

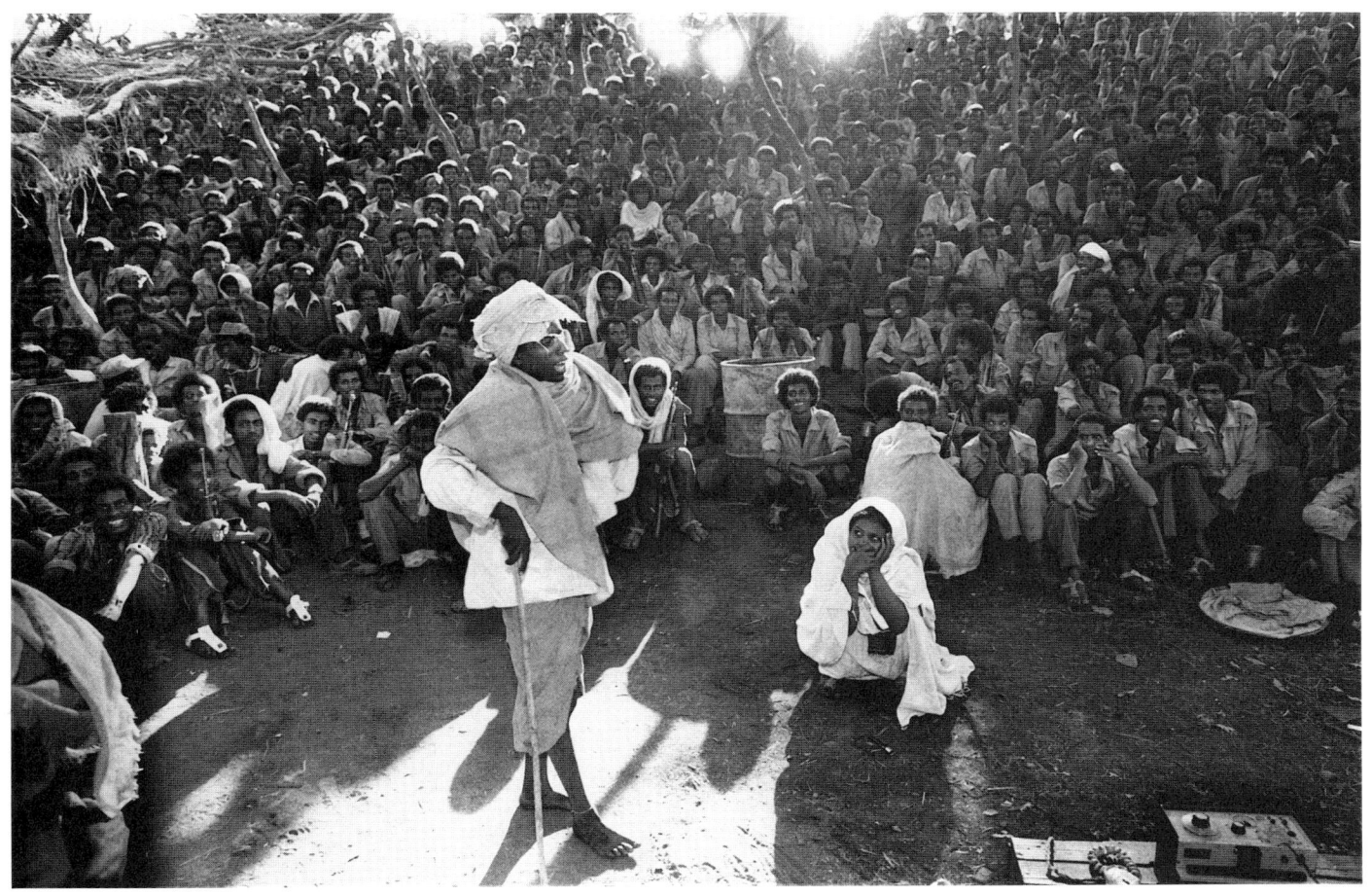

A play put on by the TPLF on the theme of
women's roles. Plays like this aim to
entertain, as well as to provoke discussion
about social issues.

Eritrea forms the northernmost strip of Ethiopia, along the Red Sea coast. It is more arid than most of Ethiopia, and rainfall in recent years has been calamitously low. Twenty-five years of war, since Haile Selassie annexed Eritrea as part of Ethiopia, have disrupted life and agriculture. Like the Tigrayans, the Eritreans have had virtually nobody to turn to but themselves. Official aid donors – the United Nations and the governments of rich countries – feel obliged to channel their aid through Addis Ababa, but independent voluntary organizations are caught in a dilemma. If they operate in Eritrea, as some do, they can be accused of political bias and of propping up a rebel army. If they don't, as equally some do not, they are accused of failing the needy.

Throughout this century, Eritrea's agricultural development has been hindered by outside forces. During the 52 years of colonial rule, the best land was taken over first by the Italians and then by the British for the production of export crops. Even then, the province was not self-sufficient in food. Since the war with Ethiopia began, hundreds of thousands of peasants have fled their land and taken refuge in the Sudan. Many of those who have stayed have seen their land repeatedly bombed, destroying crops and fodder grass.

In any war zone, long-term planning is impossible. Nonetheless, priorities can be chosen, and in Eritrea the overriding need is to increase the food production of the peasants. Agricultural development practice in Eritrea concentrates on giving a little training to a lot of people, collective use of land and resources, and the provision of seeds and elementary tools such as hoes to peasant farmers. The drought has prompted the large-scale movement of people into the Sudan, headed for the relief camps. The Eritrean Relief Association has had some success in moving food aid from the Sudan into the villages, which the Tigrayans were initially unable to do for lack of roads.

Eritrea

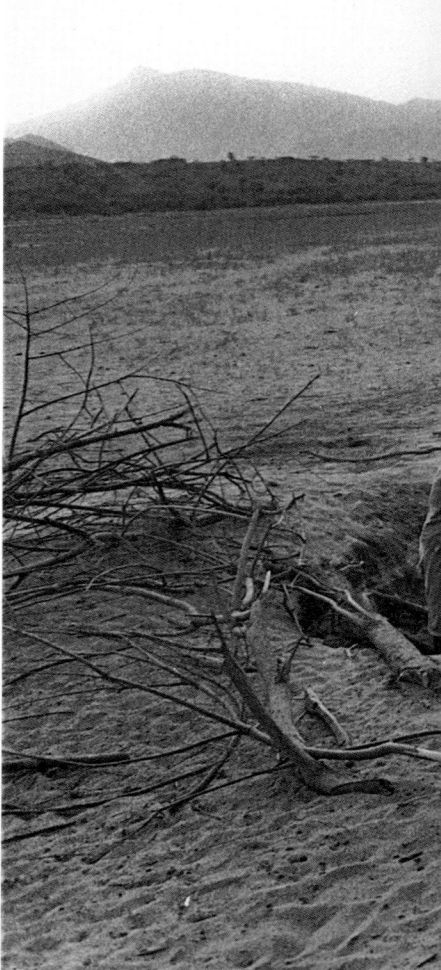

Nomads in northern Eritrea struggle to maintain their way of life in spite of war and drought. Here, they water their animals from a well in a dry river bed.

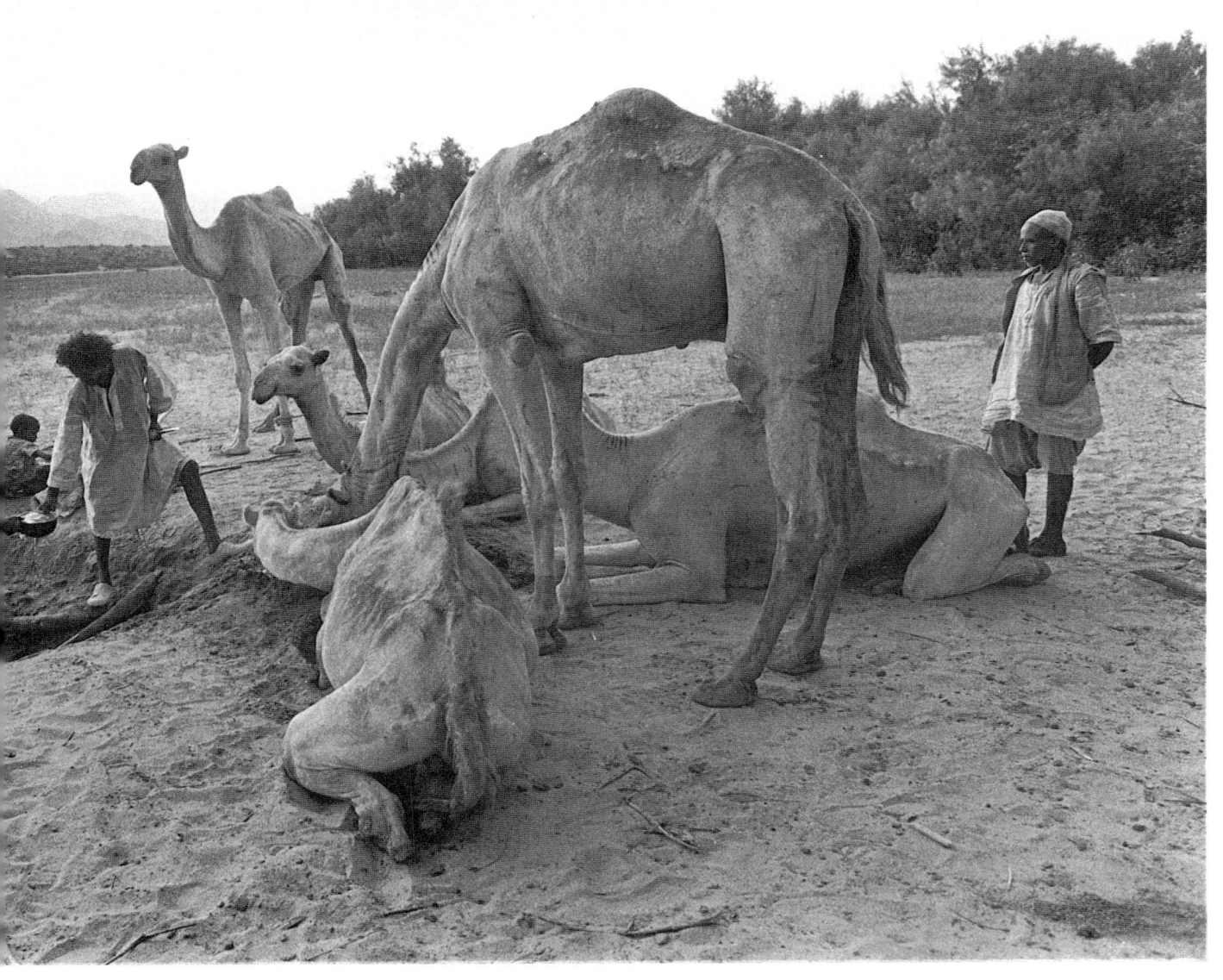

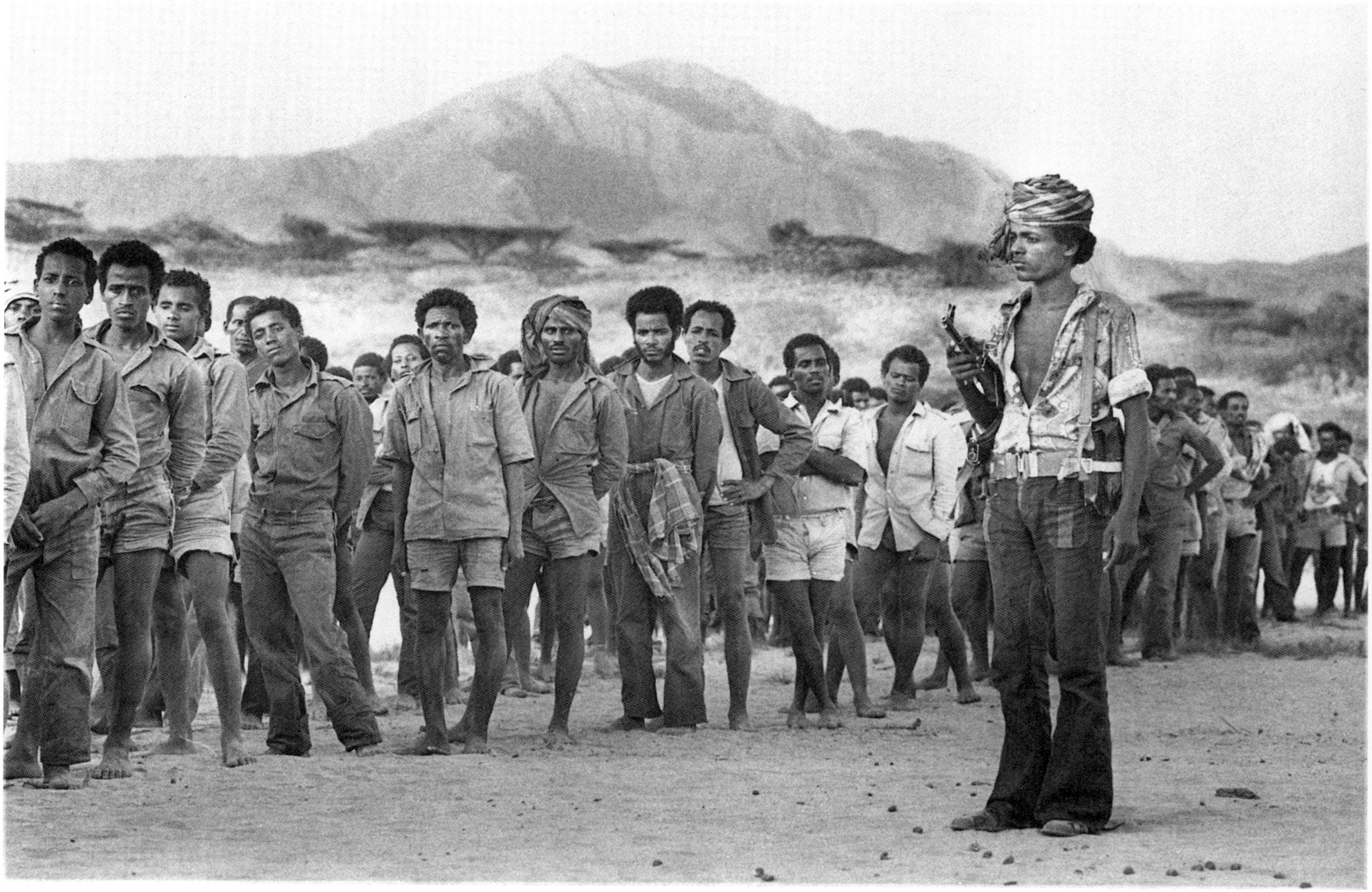

After a 25-year war of independence, the
Eritrean Peoples' Liberation Front (EPLF)
hold most of Eritrea, except for the major
towns. Here, conscripted Ethiopian
soldiers surrender to the EPLF during an
army offensive.

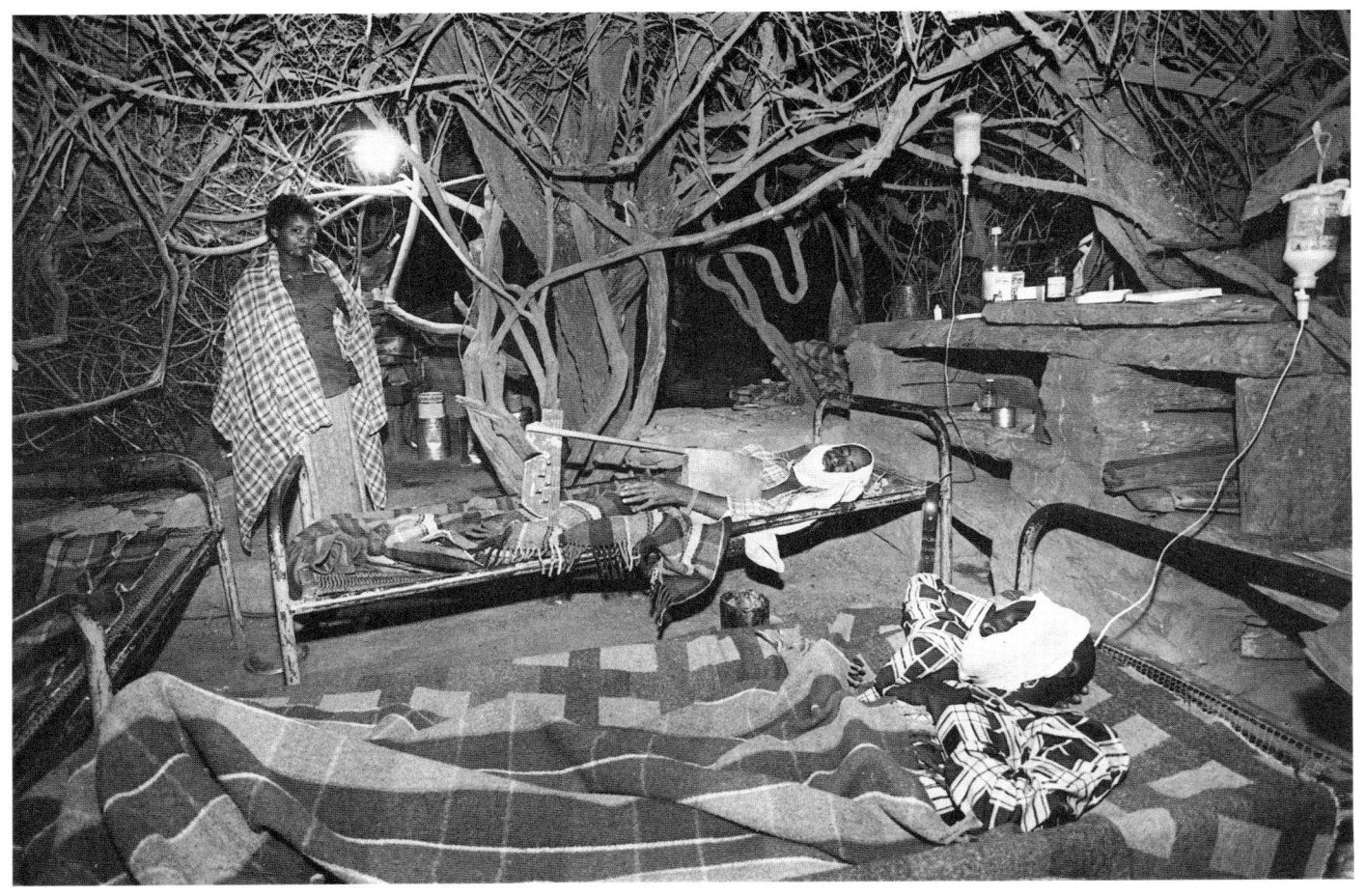

An outdoor ward for wounded fighters at
the central hospital in the EPLF's base area.

Health care

The Eritreans are also developing their own health care system. Malaria, tuberculosis and bilharzia are endemic, and average life expectancy is put at 29, compared to the Ethiopian average of 46 years. A network of hospitals has been established mainly designed to cope with the aftermath of battle. The hospitals are mobile and, to minimize the risk of aerial attack, are camouflaged by being dug into hillsides. Some wards are outdoors, hidden under trees. They cater not only for the war-wounded but also for civilians who fall into their 'catchment area', the sick people who can make the journey to the hospital.

At the same time, the Eritreans are trying to establish a village-level health care system which promotes prevention rather than cure but is also capable of administering basic treatment. The most difficult people to reach are the nomads, always on the move and culturally sceptical about the value of modern medicine. Mobile health workers visit nomad encampments on foot or by camel, and carry with them basic supplies such as essential drugs and dressings. Small clinics in the settled areas are backed up by village health committees which aim to involve the whole community in taking responsibility for hygiene, sanitation and water collection. The same strategy is being attempted by neighbouring Sudan and rests on the assumption that even poor communities can take most of the responsibility for their own physical well-being, if helped by the spread of basic information about hygiene, nutrition and a supply of essential drugs. In response to a chronic shortage of drugs and equipment, which are almost invariably expensive and imported, Eritrea has developed its own drug manufacture system, producing cheap generic antibiotics and vaccines with imported raw materials.

In both Eritrea and Tigray, war has the effect both of propelling development

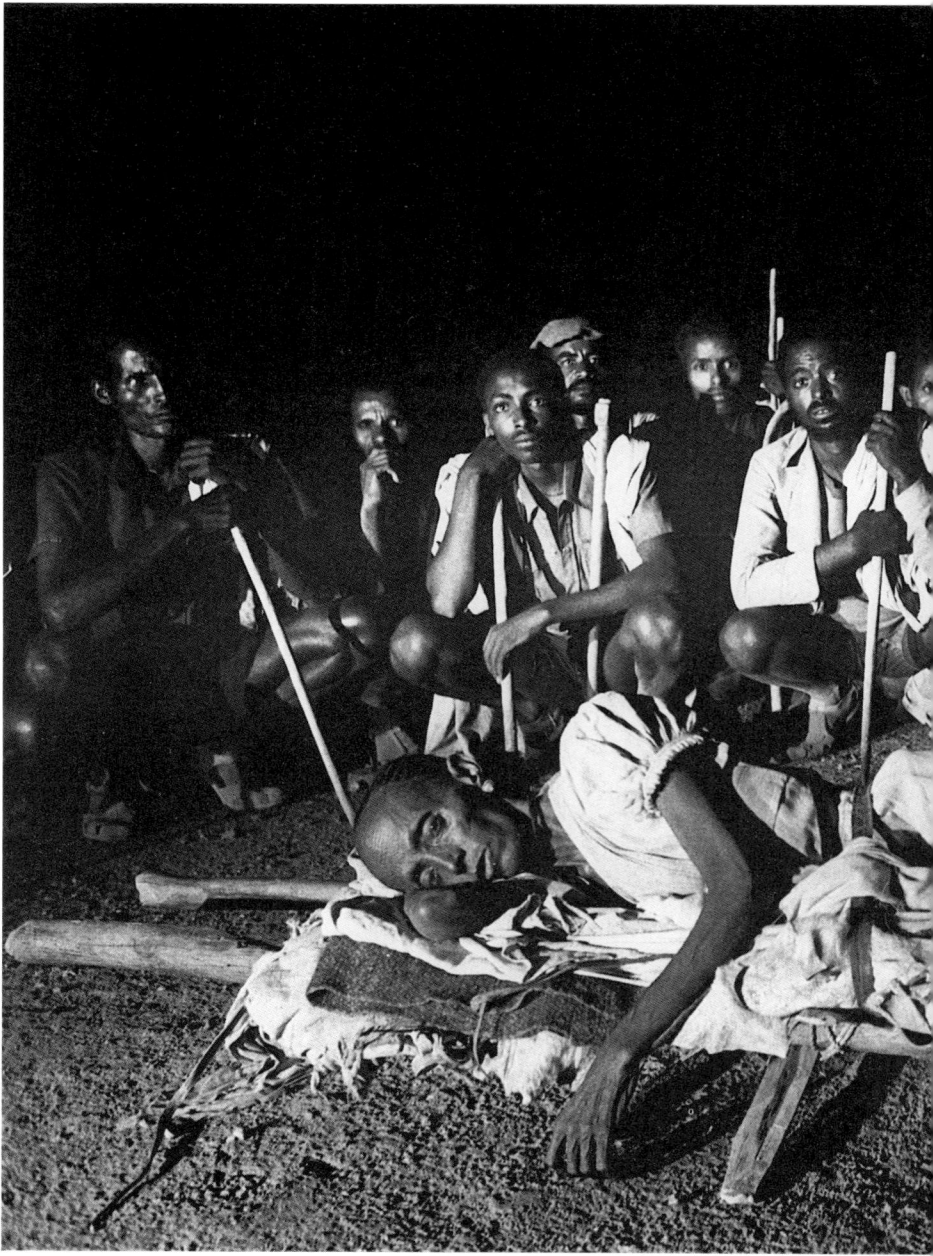

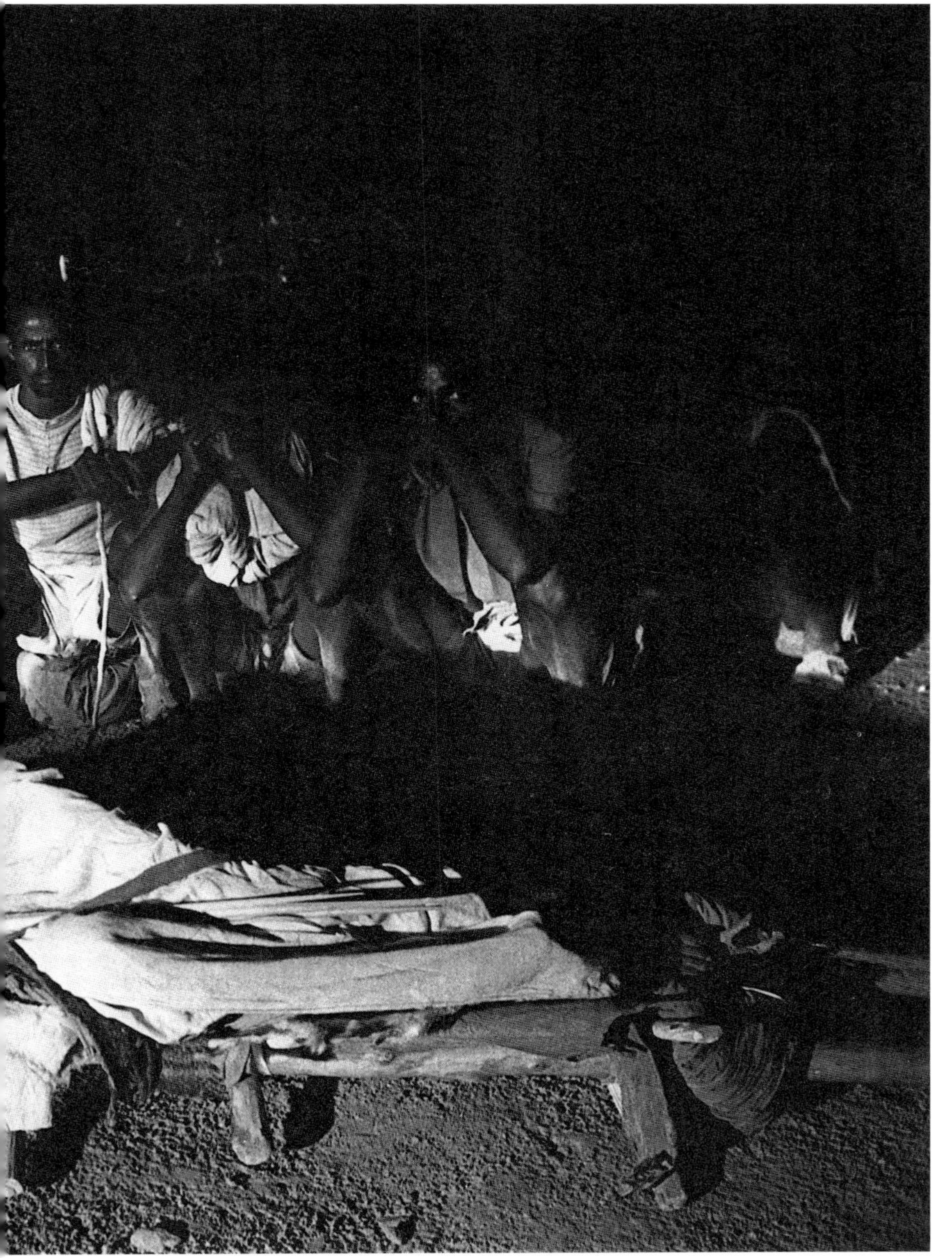

A woman being carried to hospital by men from her village.

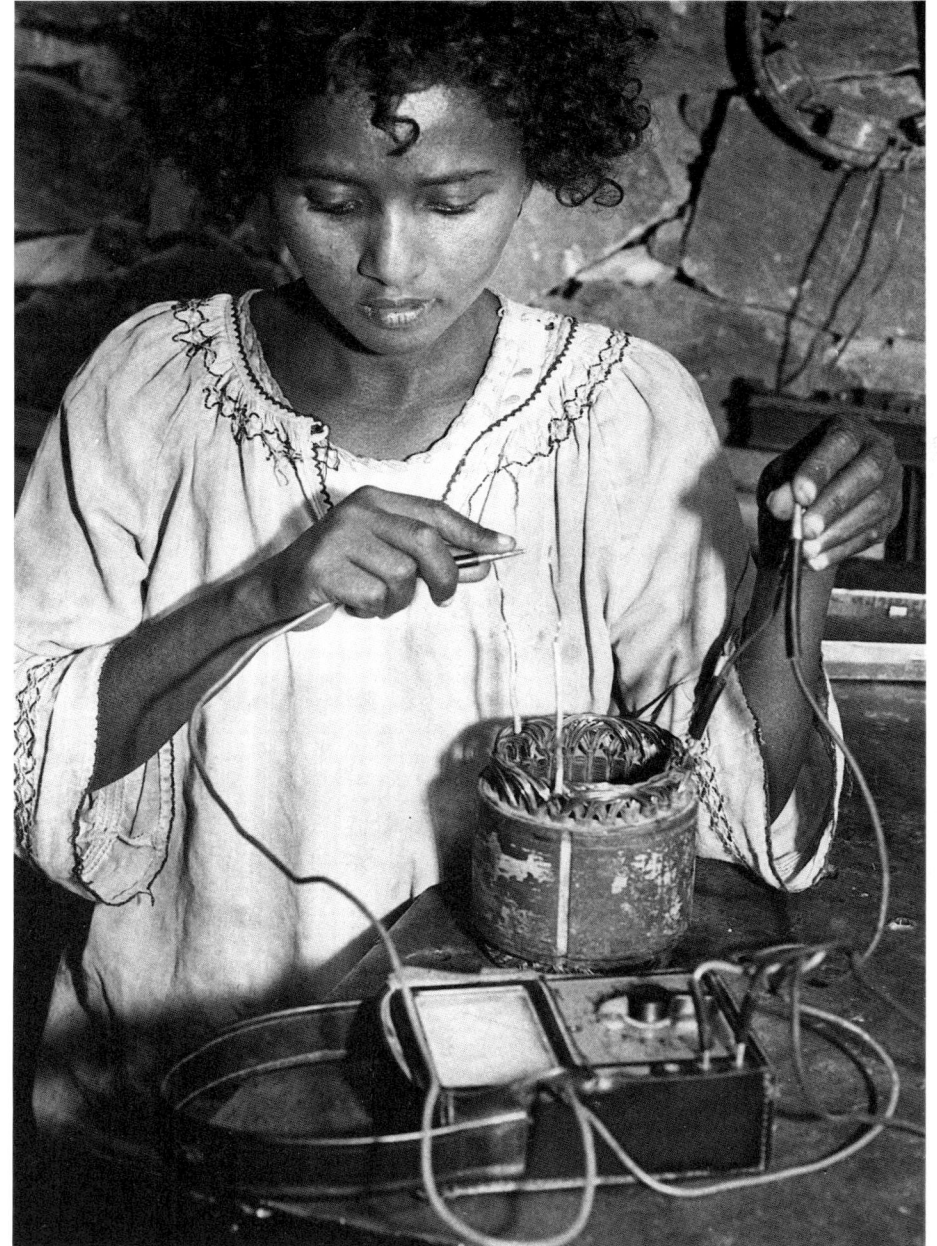

88

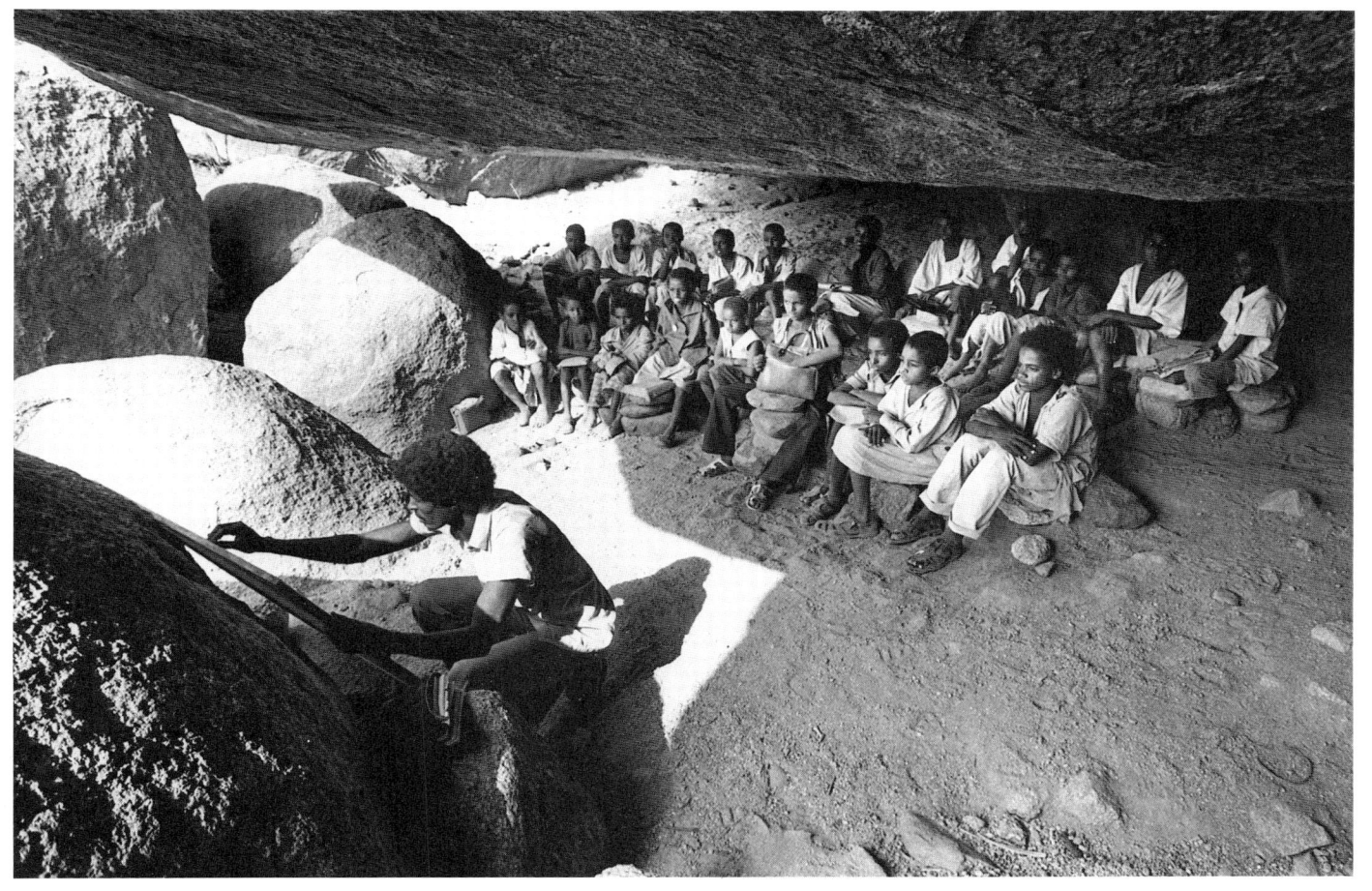

This class is being held under a rock
because of the ever-present risk of air
attack.

forward – through widespread commitment to a common cause and a de facto state of self-reliance – and of destroying many of the advances made. The large and successful irrigation project at Shawata in Tigray, for instance, is highly visible from the air and has been bombed. Likewise, many Tigrayan village clinics, often built by people who were receiving medical attention for the first time in their lives, have been destroyed. Hundreds of young Eritrean fighters have lost limbs in the war, but gained education. Many advances have been made, but the destructive effects of the wars have left thousands dead and many more lives in ruin.

Education

In many parts of Africa, one long fingernail is still the symbol of someone who has passed through the education system and therefore does no manual work. Breaking that fingernail and all it represents would signify the dismantling of the education systems set up by the colonial powers, which hinged on the creation of small educated elites. The Eritrean Peoples' Liberation Front, with their stated aim of egalitarian democracy have a mass literacy campaign underway. As part of their education, the students help in the local clinic, work on the communal land, and perform plays for discussion by the village. Education is well-integrated with village life and is not the preserve of boys from rich families.

An astonishing system of informal 'technical colleges' has been established in Eritrea, held in concealed underground workshops or classes under rocks. The 25-year-old war has necessitated the development of skills such as radio and watch repair, truck maintenance and metal-work, to service the fighters. With the struggle as their motivating force, several hundred Eritreans, men and women, have acquired technical skills which have wide-ranging application and which will be useful to the society when the war finally ends. This trained workforce would be the envy of many an African state trying to establish the same type of personnel through the educational structures of peacetime.

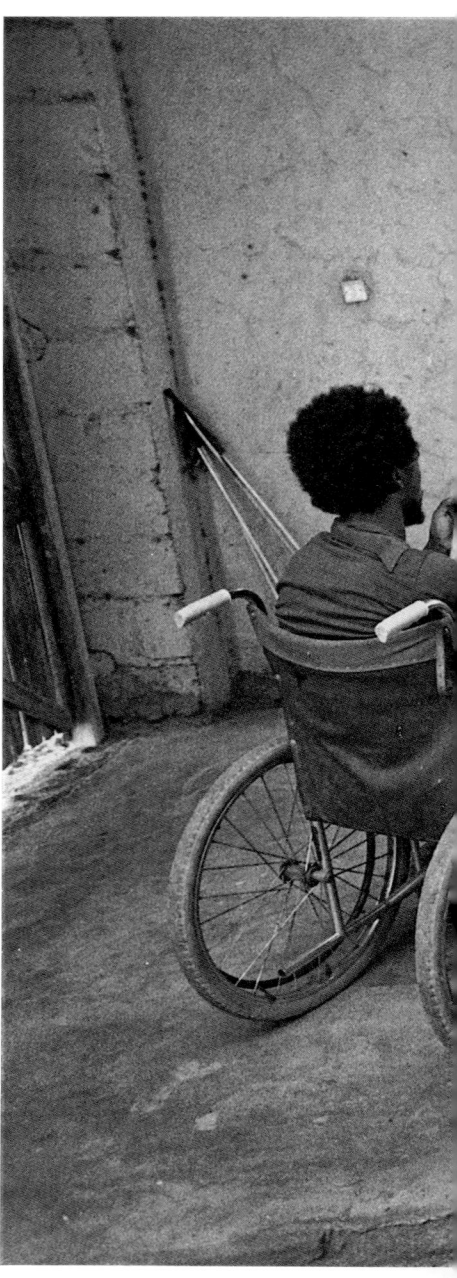

Ex-fighters at a rehabilitation centre in Sudan, run by the Eritrean Relief Association (ERA).

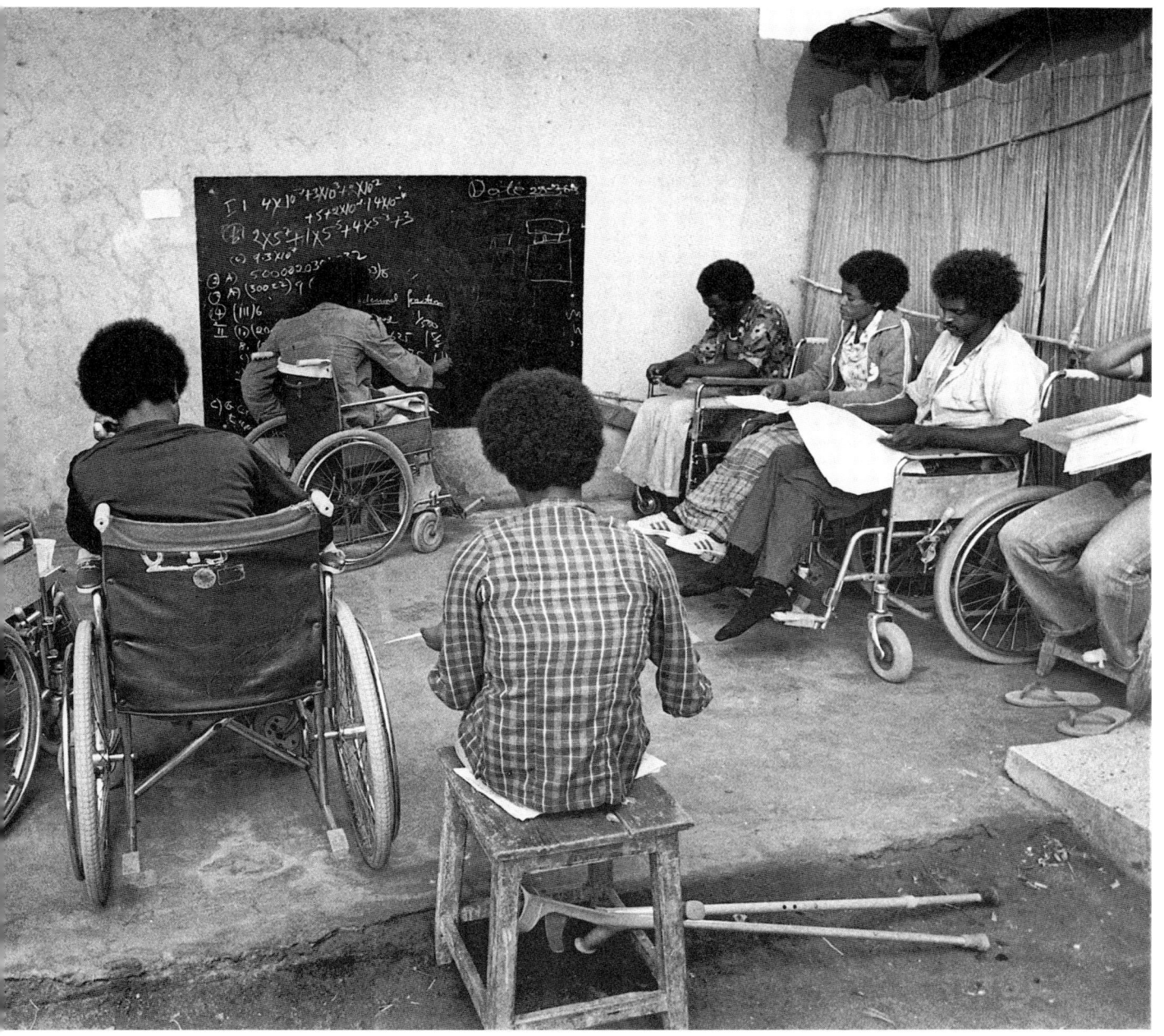

Famine has forced us to recognize that aid from rich countries over the last decade did not help the position of Africa's poorest people when drought struck. But the west is also realizing that drought and famine are not synonymous – that drought only leads to famine when families have no reserves to fall back upon. What are the major international donors, and the countries concerned, doing to halt the decline that has left the herdsmen and peasant farmers without their traditional safety net? Until recently, not much. The philosophy behind agricultural development has been to help countries boost their national incomes by growing more cash crops. Yet the international market price for these crops, so often grown at the expense of food crops, has been falling. African countries have got deeper and deeper into debt, and several states now need more than their entire national revenue just to pay the interest on their debts. Caught in this kind of vicious circle, there is little Africa can do to break the pattern.

Emergency aid to Africa during the current famine has been swift and generous. But this type of aid can never be more than a bandage on the wound. It will not stop the bleeding. That can only be done through development.

The distinguishing feature of the development taking place in both Eritrea and Tigray is that it has been initiated and carried out by the peasants themselves, in some cases with assistance from western donors. The same self-determination underlies most successful development projects in other parts of Africa, and points the way for the future of aid. But for such an approach to be possible, the current economic pressures on African governments must be eased.

What is needed is a major initiative from the industrialized countries to reform the whole structure of trade and aid. International assistance should indeed concentrate far more on food production. Rural development programmes should be geared towards the small-scale farmer. But at the same time the crippling debt burden must be eased, so that debtor countries no longer get further into debt just in order to meet interest payments on existing loans. Furthermore, commodity agreements should be overhauled to ensure that the poor countries get a better price for the raw materials they produce.

It's asking a lot – nothing less than major changes in the world's economic system. But unless these things happen, we are not leaving African governments with any choice. They will continue to ignore the needs of the bulk of their populations, aided and abetted by western donors – and the harrowing face of famine will go on haunting us.

New directions

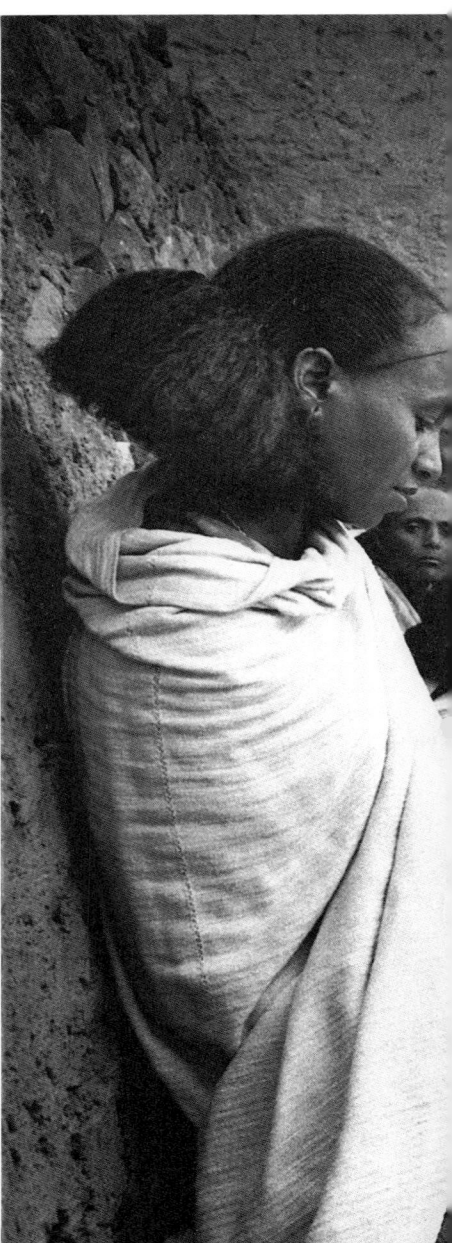

A women's association meeting at Abi Adi in central Tigray.

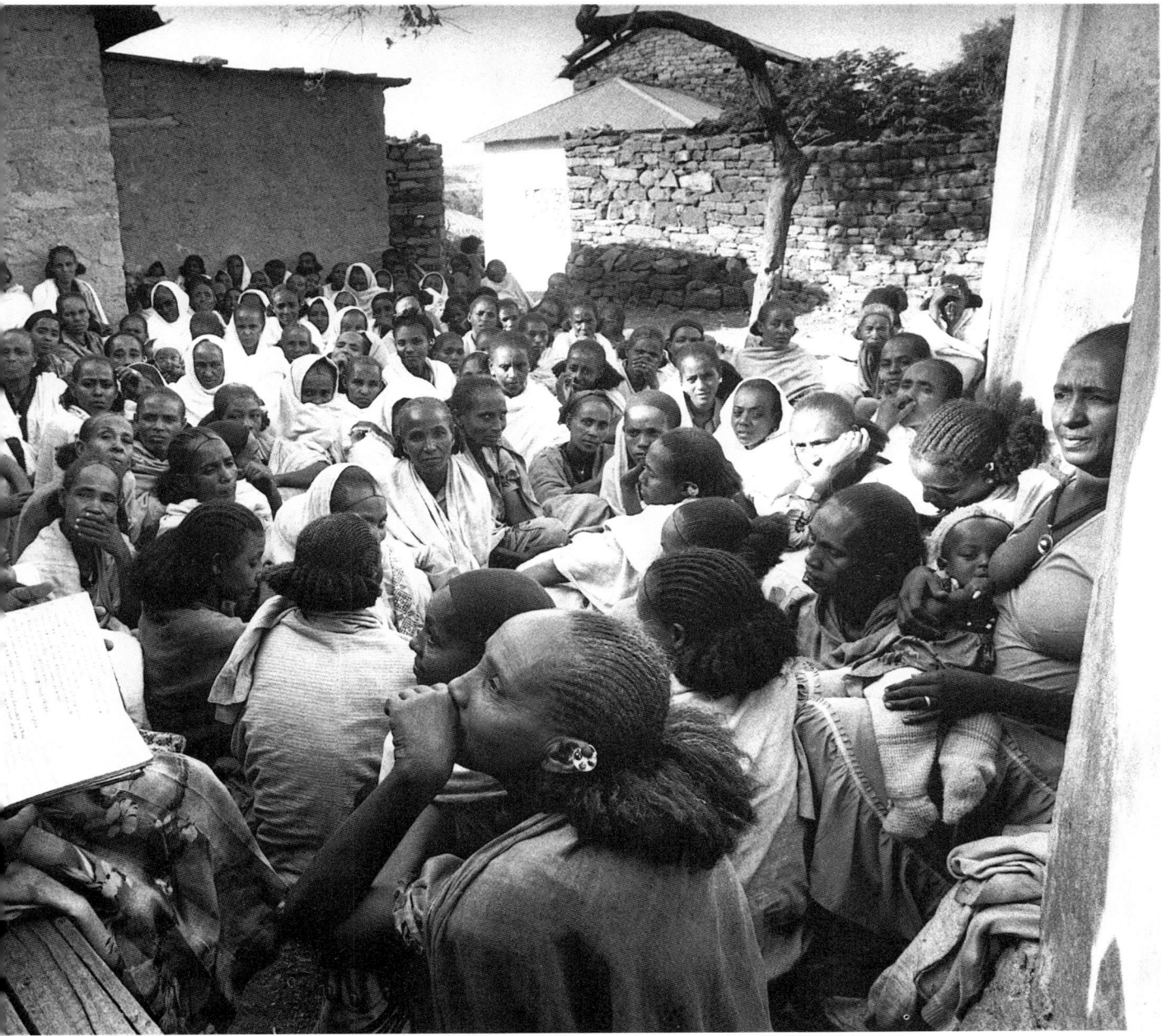

The Sahel
Richard W. Frankie and Barbara H. Chasin, *Seeds of Famine*, Allenheld Universe: New York 1980.
Nigel Twose, *Why the Poor Suffer Most*, Oxfam: Oxford 1985.

The Horn
'Conflict in the Horn of Africa', in *Review of African Political Economy*, No. 30, Sheffield 1984.

Eritrea
Basil Davidson, Lionel Cliffe and Bereket Habte Selassie (eds), *Behind the War in Eritrea*, Spokesman: Nottingham 1982.
James Firebrace with Stuart Holland, *Never Kneel Down*, Spokesman: Nottingham 1984.

Tigray
James Firebrace and Gale Smith, *The Hidden Revolution*, War on Want: London 1982.

The Environment
E. Eckholm, *Down to Earth*, Pluto Press: London 1982 (o.p.).
Allan Grainger, *Desertification*, Earthscan: London 1982.

Aid/Development
Nigel Twose, *Cultivating Hunger*, Oxfam: Oxford 1985.

Independent Commission on International Humanitarian Issues, *Famine: A Man-made Disaster*, Pan: London 1985.
Frances Moore Lappe and Joseph Collins, *Food First*, Souvenir Press: London 1980 and Institute for Food and Development Policy: San Francisco 1979.
Teresa Hayter and Catharine Watson, *Aid: Rhetoric and Reality*, Pluto Press: London 1985.
Cheryl Payter, *World Bank: A Critical Analysis*, Monthly Review Press: New York 1982.

94

FURTHER READING

In the refugee camps of Sudan the Tigrayans hold on to their culture in any way they can. Here in Safawa camp, a class of young children are chanting the alphabet in their national language, Tigrinya.

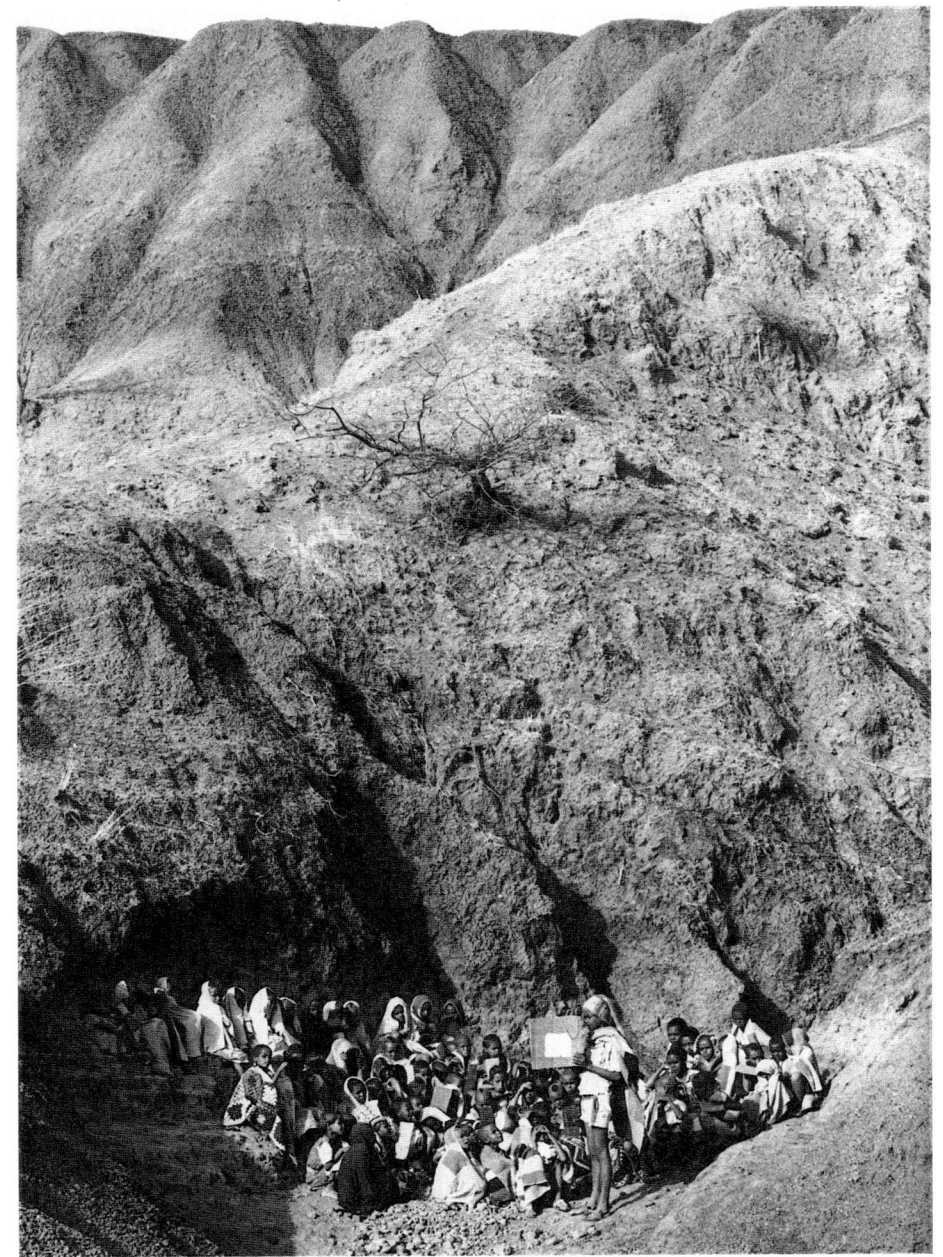

The following aid agencies contributed financially to the generation of material for this book. The views expressed are not necessarily those of the agencies. Write to them for information about their work.

CAFOD, Catholic Fund for Overseas Development, 2 Garden Close, Stockwell Road, London SW9, UK.

Christian Aid, PO Box 1, London SW9 8BH, UK.

Methodist Church Division of Social Responsibility, World Development Fund, 1 Central Buildings, Westminster, London SW1H 9NH, UK.

OXFAM, 274 Banbury Road, Oxford OX2 7DZ, UK.

SCIAF, Scottish Catholic International Fund, 43 Greenhill Road, Rutherglen, Glasgow G73 2SW, Scotland.

Trocaire – Irish Catholic Agency for World Development, 169 Booterstown Avenue, Blackrock, Co. Dublin, Republic of Ireland.

United Nations Association Trust, 3 Whitehall Court, London SW1A 2EL, UK.

War on Want, 3 Castles House, 1 London Bridge Street, London SE1, UK.

AID AGENCIES

Since 1979, Mike Goldwater has been a freelance photographer documenting international issues, including the effects of Agent Orange defoliant in Vietnam, conflict in Central America, and famine and civil war in Africa. He is a member of the London-based agency 'Network Photographers'.

Nigel Twose worked for Oxfam in the Sahel from 1979–83. His book *Why the Poor Suffer Most* investigates the harmful effects of development aid. He is currently working with Euro Action Acord, an international grouping of non-governmental organisations which fund development work in Africa.

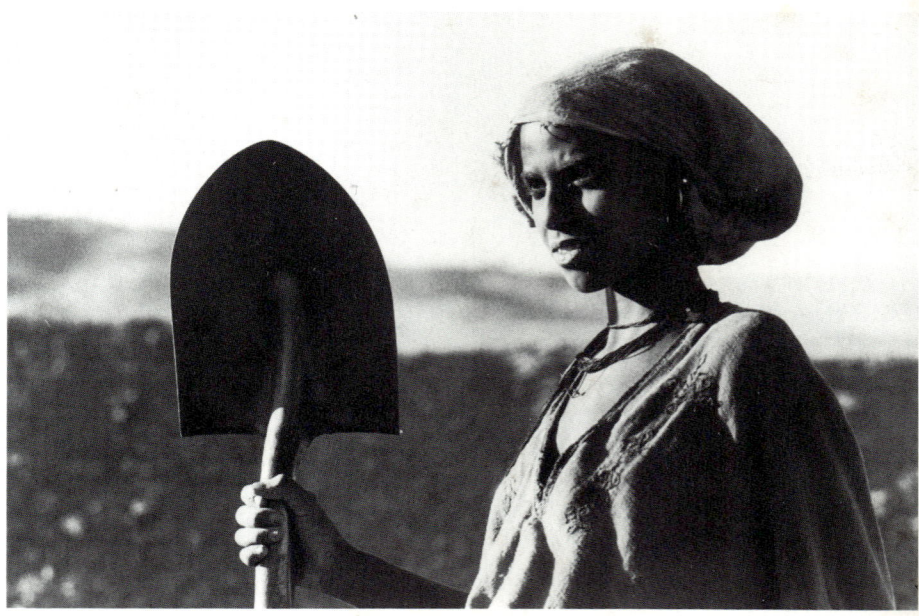